Special praise for *From Bagels to Buddha*

"Dr. Hollis has found a humorous and shockingly honest way to follow the surrender process toward freedom. Her travels to distant lands and studies with a variety of mentors shows the self-acceptance that can be achieved by turning toward and opening up, instead of turning away and tightening. With that process comes a more mindful relationship with food."

Shinzen Young
Author of *The Science of Enlightenment*
Director of Vipassana Support International

. . .

"A fabulous piece of writing. Like a descent into Hell, which turns out to be Heaven, once you get there. The idea of going there scares me, I have to say; but I might be persuaded . . . ."

Dr. Polly Howells, LCSW
Brooklyn, NY

. . .

"Dr. Judi Hollis, in a very creative, challenging, and readable way, provides us with a connection to our real bodies and our deeper souls and spirits."

Fr. Richard Rohr, OFM
Founding Director of Center for Action and Contemplation
Author of *Everything Belongs, Things Hidden,* and *The Naked Now*

. . .

"What a wonderful journey. Judi Hollis really captured her inner and outer experiences . . . and so vividly that I felt I was there."

Laura Beecher, PhD
Port Washington, NY

. . .

"With the humor that can only come from one who's been there, Dr. Judi Hollis takes us with her as she goes *From Bagels to Buddha*—the quest for a spiritual life for those who once looked for enlightenment in the bakery aisle."

Victoria Moran
Author of *Fit from Within* and *The Love-Powered Diet*

FROM

BAGELS

TO

BUDDHA

FROM
BAGELS
TO
BUDDHA

How I Found My Soul and Lost My Fat

JUDI HOLLIS, PhD

CENTRAL RECOVERY PRESS

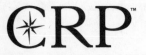

CENTRAL RECOVERY PRESS

CENTRAL RECOVERY PRESS

Central Recovery Press (CRP) is committed to publishing exceptional materials addressing addiction treatment, recovery, and behavioral healthcare topics, including original and quality books, audio/visual communications, and web-based new media. Through a diverse selection of titles, we seek to contribute a broad range of unique resources for professionals, recovering individuals and their families, and the general public.

For more information, visit www.centralrecoverypress.com.

Central Recovery Press, Las Vegas, NV 89129

Publisher: Central Recovery Press
            3321 N. Buffalo Drive
            Las Vegas, NV 89129

17 16 15 14 13 12   1 2 3 4 5

ISBN-13: 978-1-936290-81-9 (paper)
ISBN-10: 1-936290-81-2
ISBN-13: 978-1-936290-89-5 (e-book)

Publisher's Note: This is a memoir, a work based on fact recorded to the best of the author's memory. Central Recovery Press books represent the experiences and opinions of their authors only. Every effort has been made to ensure that events, institutions, and statistics presented in our books as facts are accurate and up-to-date. To protect their privacy, the names of some of the people and institutions in this book have been changed.

© Author photo courtesy of Taylor Sherrill.

Cover design and interior layout by Sara Streifel, Think Creative Design

Dedicated to the memory of my mother
for all the love, laughs, and lunacy that molded me
into the powerful, resilient woman I am today,
and to the spiritual midwives who melted my armor
so I could bend and savor the essentials.

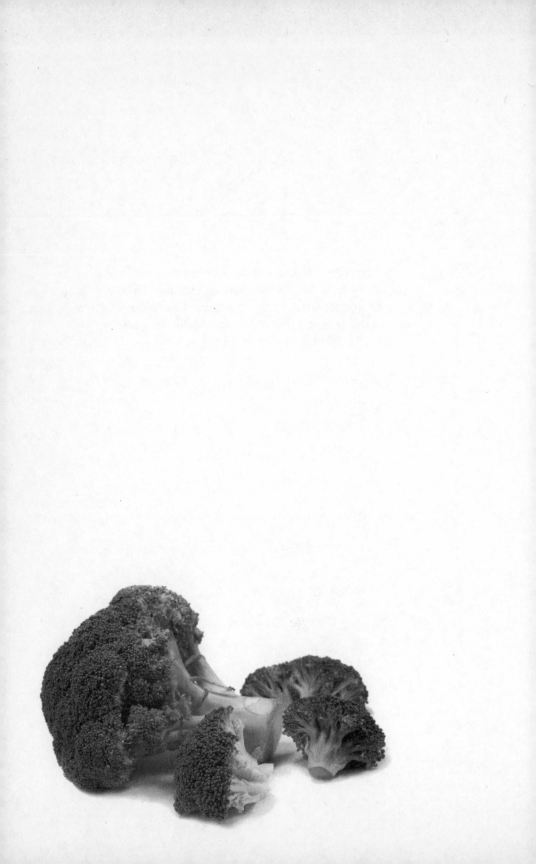

Contents

Acknowledgments

I can never repay my debt to the countless monks, teachers, mentors, sponsors, fellow wounded healers, and friends who have helped me trudge the path to self-acceptance and care. Those include Beverly R, Elaine P, Muriel Z, Arlyn R, and Kat G.

I've also been supported in this journey by my goddess group in New York—Catherine Boyer, Laura Beecher, Polly Howells, Marta Elders, Marianne Schottenfeld, and Susan Bogas. My "spooks" group in Palm Springs guides my path with wise ladies too numerous to mention. A great spiritual midwife, Elizabeth Stephenson, has been a constant source of excitement, fun, fantasy, and whimsy. I'm even now using her super-spiritual name for higher power, GGATI (God, Goddess, All That Is).

My writing has been nursed so patiently by Ray "Rusty" Straight, Deborah Herman, and my editors at Central Recovery Press, Nancy Schenck and Helen O'Reilly. My assistant, Jeff Hughes, has also helped with countless Internet and computer glitches that eventually taught us more than we ever wanted to learn. (A lot like the spiritual path.)

The most profound blessing found on this path has been my beloved lifetime companion, Henry Kaplan, who senses all the right moves and guides while adapting, cherishes while provoking, and loves me as much as I love him. His irreverence keeps me humble, alive, and open. Definitely a tastier morsel than any bagel.

Preface

"Howd-ja-doit?"

"Howd-ja-looz-althatwait?"

"Howd-ja-keepitoff?"

That's always what I'm asked.

Most people just want to know, "Whadjeet?"

They think it's only about the food.

When I opened the nation's first eating disorders unit in 1975 in Los Angeles, every new patient was contemplating an inpatient admission because he or she couldn't stop eating compulsively. Naturally, the greatest interest was focused on that most treasured love object: *the food plan*.

Of course, to lose weight and keep it off, you have to know a lot about food. Most of my patients were already amateur nutritionists. Like me, they had read it all and done it all. None of us was fat for lack of trying to lose weight. I had fought my obesity since childhood, and had gained and lost thousands of pounds. At age eight, I was taken to a specialist. We prayed for a thyroid problem that could be beaten with white pills. My mother held my hand as the doctor put me in stirrups and checked for pregnancy. It was the start of a lifetime of failed answers from Western medicine. I never returned for a GYN exam until I was twenty-two and truly pregnant.

Hoping for some magic fix kept me fat. There were no chemical or hormonal imbalances.

No such luck.

I just loved to eat.

I once asked my mother about a picture of me at age five standing on the dusty, coal-covered porch on Scranton's South Side. "Why'd you let me gorge myself with a corncob in each hand?"

Mom answered, "You just loved to eat. You were always hungry. I'd give you dinner and you'd say, 'Mommy, I want more.'"

I know today that I was ravenously hungry for a spiritual connection not to be found in food.

My "more" mantra has now become almost four decades of giving up *more* for the satisfaction of *enough*. I'm now enough. Life is enough. Today I get enough to eat.

At age twelve I started dieting for my senior prom, which ultimately I went to fat, asked as a mercy date because I was the prom chairperson. Being fat, however, didn't totally wreck my dating career since I had "such a pretty face" and was wild enough to date ne'er-do-wells and "lesser companions"—men I wouldn't take out in public. During my early career as a drug addiction counselor, I even dated a few patients. These guys were hip, slick, and cool and knew how to make a fat girl feel sexy. During my first round of Weight Watchers, I had a crush on a drug counselor. I told him I wouldn't go out with him until I "hit goal weight." He went back to drugs before I got there. There was always something.

I eventually became a nine-time loser at Weight Watchers; I lost each time, and I was later hired as a consultant. When I tried acupuncture, the needles fell out of my ears. Protein drinks and restrictive diets worked until I ended those forays and binged. The truth is that most of us are expert "dieters" for as long as we stay on the diets.

All diets work. Take your pick. Mark Twain said, "It's easy to stop smoking. I've done it hundreds of times." But how do we *stay* stopped? What does one do when firm resolve lessens and eating excess food seems the best alternative?

We eat. And, as overeaters, we eat a lot. And we usually regain more weight than we lost.

For permanent weight loss, I had to first learn that there is more to life than four ounces of protein, a cup of vegetables, and ten laps around the pool. And there is more to beating the weight game than intellect. I certainly was smart enough to stay thin. But to stay at a healthy weight, knowing stuff is only part of the equation. The permanent weight-loss goal lies somewhere beyond reason. In fact, I have found that the smarter we are, the more trouble we have surrendering to spirit. I had to surrender to my spiritual instincts. Transcendence cannot be cooked up from a recipe. The spiritual path is personal and precarious. We must first hit our own wall, lean into it, stay awake, accept help, get honest, own our dark side, live at risk, forgive softly, laugh gratefully, give generously, and trust the body's still voice to tell us how. Then we'll each find personal wisdom in our own Buddha nature.

A client once told me, "I get up in the morning and my head mugs me." Being in your own head is like being caught behind enemy lines.

So many are now going under the knife, people are beginning to understand how hard it is to lose weight and keep it off. Most know that the statistics indicate a 98 percent failure rate for all dieters, with only 2 percent achieving lifelong, permanent weight loss. I've been in that 2 percent for more than three decades now, and I'd like to expand that slim margin by inviting you in.

We've all read about our national overeating epidemic. Americans have a super-sized appetite for fast foods, but that's not our only problem. Our national girth has more to do with our spiritual connections—how we live, how we think, how we fight, how we love, how we die. We compete and strive to win. We overwork, overplay, overthink, and then eat mindlessly and ravenously. Genetics might load the gun, but environment pulls the trigger.

The journey is not a battle, but a surrender—a surrender to a more spiritual way of living. However, the spiritual life is not for sissies. Some may think that wearing Birkenstocks or lighting incense gets them in, but one can't just look the part or go through the motions. I thought I could hang out with the "metaphysical maniacs" for six months, become my own personal guru, and then revert to self-abuse. Instead, I learned that staying thin happens not through competition, fighting, or winning, but by gently leaning in and letting go.

You might initially feel you are too smart for this "airy-fairy" stuff. I knew that my personal god of intellect had helped me to survive. After I had survived many life crises through cunning and guile, my tombstone might have read, "Nobody got the best of her." I didn't see that in some areas my brain was wired for self-abuse.

I first had to truly, truly, truly admit defeat and ask for help. Early on, I surrendered enough to ask a spiritual mentor for guidance. Initially attracted to her neat, polished, clean looks and her singsong, almost too-syrupy voice, I let her know during our first phone call, "I'm a therapist. I know a lot about addiction. I think I continue to gain weight because I am praaaabaaaaabbbblleee afraid to get thin."

She answered quietly, "Why don't you get thin, and then we'll talk about it."

Damn! Cut the wind right out of my sails. No bull. No psychobabble.

I continued, "I like everything about your weight-loss plan except the spiritual part."

She replied, "There is no spiritual *part*. My plan is a total, 100 percent, take-no-prisoners spiritual program. It *is* spiritual and nothing else."

Eventually, as you'll read here, I got it. Hopefully, you will too.

In the Passover service celebrating Moses's flight from Egypt, fathers all over the world recite a passage from the Haggadah: "This is what the Lord G-d did for *me* as he led *me* out of the land of Egypt." Even though this commemorates events from many centuries ago, we view any transit out of slavery as if it happens for us all right here and now. Freedom for any one of us can create healing for *all* of us. So instead of examples from my patients' struggles, as I had offered in previous books, I will share with you what happened for me personally. My vignettes, written over a twenty-year period, represent my continuing personal surrender process.

In my journey you will see a gentler, inward approach, one that you, too, can embrace as you travel on your own journey to surrender. You will find a personal way to give up the glommed-on, overstuffed, bloated feeling of too many bagels (metaphorically speaking), and to replace it with a free-floating, risky uncertainty. Oddly enough, as you open up and embrace that uncertainty, you won't feel as smart, but you will know and see a lot more. This is what many who follow Eastern philosophy refer to as your "Buddha nature."

Surrendering to that Buddha nature does not necessitate becoming religious. You can surrender to spiritual weight loss without believing in any deity. You can start walking the spiritual path even if your heels are digging grooves into the flooring. You can balance surrender with action, teasing out which actions are yours to take on and when it is right for you to let go. You act some. You wait some. It can be like listening to the pledge break announcer on public television: "We've got a matching donor! For every dollar you put up, our donor will provide a matching pledge." You can echo the fishermen who advise, "Pray toward heaven, but row toward shore," or the Muslim trader who warns, "Trust Allah, but tie your camel."

I will not advocate for any specific organized religion; instead, I invite you to find your own spiritual connections. Spirituality and religion are two completely different concepts. I believe, and I've heard it expressed this way, that religion is for people who fear hell, while spirituality is for those who've been there. I also believe that those who face and acknowledge the fears and admit to the horrors they've lived through and the struggles they've overcome are certainly strong enough to surrender to the spiritual path. When you acknowledge feeling fear but stop fighting it, you will enter a new and stronger phase of growth. You feel the fear, but do it anyway.

None of us is ready until we're ready. I had to weigh 222 pounds before I asked for help. I'd been a pioneer in addiction counseling since 1967 when I first worked for New York's Mayor Lindsay in the Addiction Services Agency. I went on to graduate school, consulted with the US Navy's alcoholism programs, and continued to develop early-addiction treatment programs throughout Southern California. I counseled thousands of others while I continued to gorge and binge.

Eventually, I surrendered over and over and over again. As I achieved en-*lighten*-ment, emotionally and spiritually, I lightened up the outsides, physically and behaviorally.

To maintain my seventy-pound weight loss for more than three decades, I had to learn a lot about surrender. Spiritual mentors taught me new ways to act so I could feel better about myself. As a result of "doing the right thing," I stopped punishing myself with excess food. As an overeater, I had confused nurturance with punishment.

While finding the spiritual path, I often didn't get my own way. I had to throw away my rule book. Each new time I gave up my self-will was just as difficult as the first time. Of course, the most difficult early surrender was following direction on a food plan. Once overeating was curtailed, all the other surrenders were that much more difficult. There was no convenient crutch of excess food to help me weather the changes. Many times I was instructed to do things totally against my instincts. For example, as a practitioner in addiction treatment who had been advised by spiritual mentors, I knew it was the right thing to refuse to bail my husband out of jail. Even though my head knew it was the right course, my whole body shook as I put down the phone receiver after I told him, "I just can't come." Then, before my first-ever television appearance, I quaked in fear in my size-24 flowered muumuu, and said I couldn't do it. A spiritual mentor advised, "Suit up and show up and do what's put in front you." And then, after being attacked on a high-profile afternoon talk show, insisting I would not go back, I listened as my mentor directed, "It's not your show, and it's not about you. You have a responsibility to deliver a message." When a jealous psychiatrist stole my first treatment program and plagiarized my early notes for *Fat Is a Family Affair,* I was again counseled not to sue, but to let it go. My own survival was more important. Each surrender I embraced brought more weight loss.

Most of my early surrenders were in situations involving attacks from the outside. Each time, I gave up my conniving, manipulative, controlling responses to stand with quiet integrity, allowing the universe to yield its results. I ultimately found that in seeking a spiritual solution, it didn't serve me well to pick apart the actions of others. What benefited me the most was when I examined my own behavior and admitted my own shortcomings.

It was only after many years of practice that I was ready for the biggest surrender of all: the surrender to self. No longer was the external world menacing, but I faced a struggle from within— accepting myself as a fallible human being.

I invite you to travel with me as I journey from a Buddhist monastery in California to basement detox centers in New York, to Oprah's favorite spa resort in Arizona, to Peruvian mountaintops, to a Native American sweat lodge outside Santa Fe, to a Russian bathhouse on New York's Lower East Side, to yoga and massage centers in India, to the highlands of Burma (now called Myanmar), and ultimately back home to the Big Apple.

You won't have to travel to strange lands to have your own, equally exotic, personal journey. Excesses of bagels, or whatever your food of choice may be, clog up your psyche, offering a false sense of security, a false-bottomed foundation, which keeps you feeling glued but in the end leaves you screwed. I invite you on a journey to give up that heavy, overstuffed feeling for the powerful emptiness of your own free-floating, Buddha nature. Some of these ideas were set down by Eastern holy men thousands of years ago. Some were instituted by two drunks in Akron, Ohio, more than half a century ago. Offered here is a synthesis to provide an operating mode to overcome modern, chronic food obsessions.

INTRO

Obesity as a Spiritual Crisis

According to the Centers for Disease Control and Prevention (CDC), obesity affects over 33 percent of Americans—that's one-third of adults. Medical costs associated with obesity are estimated at $147 billion, and obese adults are at a higher risk for coronary heart disease, type 2 diabetes, high blood pressure, stroke, liver and gallbladder disease, and respiratory problems. In addition, obese adolescents are more likely to have prediabetes, a condition in which blood glucose levels indicate a high risk for development of diabetes. Americans are some of the fattest people on earth, gorging at elegant tables, all-you-can-eat buffets, and fast-food drive-thrus, or competing in hot dog–eating contests. We are slowly and complacently adapting to "more is not enough" as we seek excess food to cope with our lives, which speed along in overdrive. Our quest to fill that bottomless plate not only affects our health, but also takes a toll on the animals and plants with which we share our Mother Earth. Sadly, as a result, some of us vomit to escape the consequences, and some, like I did, simply overeat and accumulate excess weight.

Despite our extensive knowledge about calorie counts, food combining, pulse rates, and body fat indexes, we keep putting on more and more weight. Great and wonderful tomes have already been written that explain how cultural expectations of unnatural thinness have created this national epidemic. It may be that advertisers have contributed to the anorexia-bulimia-obesity triad, but there is more to it than the model culture, fitness crazes, heart disease, diabetes, or other food-related maladies. We are facing a spiritual crisis and are eating to quell the pain while avoiding our fears. Advertising ploys work because they address America's abundance conundrum: we have so much, and we still long for more, and yet we fear living with the consequences that come from wanting and getting more.

Fat is fear? Do you even know you are afraid? President Franklin Roosevelt addressed a fearful nation with "The only thing we have to fear is fear itself." Once the nation acknowledged that feeling, it could then face those fears and show up with courage, resolve, and pride.

Some of us thought the women's movement of the 1970s would change things, but instead women showed up acting more like men. Despite all the feminist gains, we still live in a male-oriented culture that seeks to avoid feeling fear at all costs. Striving for and competing against are now our mantras. On national television shows, we pit obese sufferers against each other. Thin viewers laugh at the contestants while the obese cry and feel further hopelessness. We tragically compete at weight loss. America's national epidemic is evidenced in the bulbous softness of our bodies, while we fear letting too much softness and kindness into our hearts. Fear, if unacknowledged, has to go somewhere. For many of us, it's piled onto our plates and eventually lands on our hips, thighs, and stomachs or waits in ambush inside our arteries.

Could it be that our national obesity crisis is based on this cultural denial? *Denial* stands for **D**on't **E**ven **N**otice **I A**m **L**ying. Rarely do we sit down to just say out loud, "I'm afraid." Acknowledging the fear doesn't mean succumbing to it. It just means you embrace who you are and what is going on in your life. The word *fear* is sometimes read as an acronym: **F**alse **E**vidence **A**ppearing **R**eal. A raunchier way to describe fear is **F**_ck **E**verything **A**nd **R**un. As you begin your personal journey as witnessed in this book, fear will come to mean **F**ace **E**verything **A**bout **R**esistance.

A Tibetan monk, who was an honored guest at a Manhattan literati party, was approached by a full-of-herself popular novelist. She asked, "So what is Buddhism, anyway?"

He smiled. "Do you want the short version or the long one?"

She replied, "The short version. It's a party, after all."

"Well, the short version is 'Pay attention.'"

Baffled by not enough information, she prodded, "Well, the long version, then."

He responded, "The long version is 'Pay attention. Pay attention. Pay attention.'"

When you practice paying attention, you will find that there is a lot more going on than you ever noticed before. When excess eating is curtailed, your senses will be heightened, and you will feel your emotions in a much deeper and more vibrant way. You will enter the spiritual dimension with a sense of awe.

Coincidences may begin to occur as you start to realize that your actions will often produce instantaneous and direct consequences. You will notice your own part in creating problems in your life, and you may find yourself watching your new, gentler behaviors with amusement. As you do things in a whole new way, your love affair with food and excess will change. Sometimes your attraction to food will be a mere shrug, as if to say, "No big deal."

I find it a great cosmic joke that most of us are impatient and intolerant individuals who have been given a body that won't lose weight on our timetable. Instead, it produces unexpected cravings, nonscheduled undulations, gaseous emissions, and clamorous noises beyond our will. Over time, I found that I would have to learn to trust that body as my conduit to spirit. I was advised early on, since I wasn't a believer and rebelled against any mention of God, to try the Quakers' concept: "God is the still, small voice within." This body of mine that seems to have a mind of its own will be my goddess, my transmitter, my dilemma, my teacher, and my karma.

Karma is what my addict patients would refer to as "What goes around comes around" and what my Bible-thumping friends would quote as "You reap what you sow." My Jewish relatives would advise that you reap your rewards here on earth in this lifetime. My existentialist professors would caution that there are always consequences, and that "not to decide is to decide." For those of us who love to eat, karma is best explained as "There is no free lunch."

It seems that many of us avoid surrender and avoid accepting how gifted and special we really are. Perhaps you might be afraid to truly live the big life intended for you. Perhaps you might be hiding under a rock, refusing to let your little light shine. As sentient beings, we are chosen to express a deep spiritual longing, what Carl Jung called a "cosmic homesickness." Buddhists explain that we seek "the Eternal." We know there is more going on than our minds can dream up. For all the Freudian, or scientific, or mechanistic thinking posited during the twentieth century, today we are suffering large-scale addiction and out-of-control obesity—our modern plague.

Many may think becoming spiritual will make them look good. They hope to achieve an angelic pose, positioning themselves above the fray. Actually, becoming spiritual may make you look worse for a while. You will truly open up an avenue to your own dark side, and you may want to hide. St. John of the Cross called such periods the "Dark Night of the Soul." Forgiving yourself may become the ultimate spiritual awakening, causing transcendence into what some twelve-steppers call "the fourth dimension."

This transcendence occurs slowly as you take an honest look at yourself. It takes time and effort and initially seems like excessive self-obsession. One addict patient told me, "My head is permanently tuned to Radio K-F-_-C-K, all me, all the time." Taking that honest look means acknowledging all your assets, as well as your liabilities, rendering you a little more humble. You might uncover motives and behaviors you find embarrassing. That embarrassment helps you become teachable. You'll learn to love your neuroses, and your quirks and foibles, as signposts indicating your next spiritual breakthrough. Until you can learn to laugh at yourself, you haven't really surrendered to the spiritual path. Eventually, self-obsession will lead to an honest appraisal of your motives and values and you'll begin thinking more of others. You might even find them interesting.

At some point, you might even feel blessed and thankful to have a food obsession. You'll see that your compulsive eating is a signal that something is wrong. It is a searchlight signaling for rescue boats. When pounds pile on, you get a clear indication that you've steered off course. What an accurate barometer. Our defects or neuroses are the signals that we are living out of sync with our true inner natures. They are our coping mechanisms to fend off fear and help us survive. Some folks never examine their true motives and needs, and instead relapse back into excesses and old behaviors. Instead of changing old responses, they retreat into familiar patterns of resentment, guilt, arrogance, and control. In the end, they binge. I wonder if they are the 98 percent of us who regain lost weight.

A spiritual life involves risk. To lose the fat risk, you must live *at risk*. This journey must be carried on with a forward momentum. You can ill afford to hang back and stay asleep. There is no escape into unconsciousness. Your soul knows. It will not allow dawdlers on the path. Staying locked in fear and inertia leads back to excessive eating. You must reach for your fate instead of a plate.

Sometimes people seek to avoid risk by running into *ana*lyzing. Looking back at when I opened the nation's first eating disorders unit, I regret that I contributed to this problem. On stage and screen I was quite vociferous about the disease concept and the similarities between overeating and other addictions. I encouraged looking at the obsessive eating problem as a medical malady. I'd seen how that approach had benefited alcoholics, addicts, and their families. It helped them stop punishing themselves. I encouraged attendance at twelve-step meetings and offered an addiction model as a course of treatment.

However, some practitioners have taken this approach too far, stopping at diagnosis and not surrendering to the spiritual path of not knowing, of having fewer succinct answers. They strongly emphasize ideas about "food addiction" and are fearful of any sugar or white flour and insist on a concept of *abstinence*. They haven't accepted that those who struggle with food obsession are given a problem that needs daily and continual renegotiation, and often the sufferers have to proceed blindly with no clear-cut answers. These practitioners fail to mention that many foods break down in the system to sugar anyway, and there are issues of timing and exercise involved with how the body processes these substances. They also fail to allow for any moderation or flexibility, not adapting food consumption to real-life situations. They are afraid of what Buddhists propose as the "middle path."

Many people can survive the big traumas of life by battening down the hatches, gliding into their ninja stance, and getting ready for the onslaught. They've grown accustomed to stress and don't feel that they deserve any peace. It's the good life that presents a variety of challenges. Most don't even know what peace looks like, or have a clue about how to be happy and content. What happens to that human fighter energy? How does one show up quietly to live an ordinary day as an average Jane?

After the initial introduction to a new way of life without excess, you need encouragement and support from someone slightly ahead of you on the path, to show you how to "keep on keepin' on." In addition to advice from experts, you need modeling and direction from those who've walked before you. They can help you to forgive yourself as well as others. That's why I encouraged attendance at twelve-step groups. I know how much people need help further down the line after the initial zeal and firm resolve wanes.

My whole purpose in developing eating-disorder units along the lines of addiction treatment was to offer overeaters an opportunity to get off their own backs. I saw that helping people acknowledge and accept that they had already tried their best would make them available to receive help from others. They weren't bad people trying to get good, but rather sick people trying to get well. I also saw the similar psychological makeup between overeaters and alcoholics/addicts, and realized that they needed similar types of group and family therapy and similar spiritual interventions. But all needed an initial surrender, and each individual must find his or her own way.

Maturity is the ability to live with unresolved problems. Living with fewer answers can help you to open up to the wonder of life. If you want to heal and grow, you must become a spiritual adult. Whether you had a battered childhood or not, whether you grew up in poverty or not, even if you were "disadvantaged" in every way, you can begin a brand-new life today. Surrender allows you to be master of your own fate.

Even if life is risky, you can walk more gently and positively, as if the outcome is already written. You do the best you can to direct your intentions toward the outcome you'd like, and then gratefully hold the results with a loose hand.

Eventually you might even be grateful for your struggles with food. Sir William Osler, an early teacher in American medicine, advised that the key to longevity was to develop a lifelong, chronic illness and focus on taking care of it. That is the purpose your food obsession serves. It keeps you awake, keeps you paying attention, and keeps you motivated for self-care—that is, *if* you keep paying attention. According to the National Weight Loss Registry, which accumulates data on those who've maintained large weight losses over time, two important behaviors show up across the board: people who weighed themselves regularly and kept some form of food journal were most successful. They remained conscious and awake.

Those of you who struggle in your relationship with food have an extremely persistent problem. You are prone to relapse and will probably revert back to compulsive eating. The only constant principle will be: get back on the horse. No matter what, each day, every day requires saddling up and getting back on that horse. Day after day after day, get back in the race. It is best to make sure you are riding in the direction the horse is going. If not, don't complain about a saddle horn up your rump.

A great spiritual leader once said, "You *be* the change you want to see in the world." It is when you take on acts of loving kindness, like saving a spider or doing your job without ego just because it needs to be done, that your actions change you. *You* get the feeling of peace and responsibility because that's what you outwardly project. *You* become what you want to be. What three things could you do differently this week in order to demonstrate the way you would like to be treated? Try it and see if you don't get back what you give out.

You may balk at my proposition that overeating represents a crisis in spiritual development. You may be like many of my patients who were avid churchgoers, organizers of many charities, dedicated to helping others, behaving in what they felt was a spiritual manner. They all looked the part, even the 600-pound father of eight who told me he could not adhere to my recommendations because he had to devote most of his free time to the church. He died in a pew.

He and many others were not able to balance self-care with overly zealous caring for others. They didn't adhere to the airline instructions to grab for your own oxygen mask before attending to your babies. They didn't honor the sacredness of their own bodies and psyches. They gave and gave and gave, then felt depleted, and filled themselves with excess. Is this you?

Or are you a person who takes on self-care as a spiritual quest? An essential part of you seeks your own lightness. You have probably spent years talking about seeking a lighter body weight. I'm suggesting a different lightness (spirituality), which, once found, will help your body contour to its proper size and heft and stay there. As my lecture career moves into its fourth decade, I meet up with people who've heard me speak many years before. Though they note that my body is still slim and healthy, they comment, "You were really hellfire and brimstone in the old days. Now, you seem so much softer." Taking an honest look at yourself and seeking compassionate understanding can often help you to soften up as well.

Please use this book as your personal fabric softener. When I initially proposed the disease concept for overeaters, it gave them permission to accept themselves and soften a little. This offered a justification to take time out of a busy life to attend self-help meetings, or a license to ask the waitress to take back the tossed salad and bring one with the dressing on the side, or a way to say "no" to a demanding family member piling on more work, or even as permission to take a legitimate thirty-minute lunch break. Attending to their malady made them stronger people. When you accept that you have a disease, you take yourself seriously, and you ask for the same consideration from others.

Walking the planet more softly and developing openness and lightness and a more inquiring mind is a fundamental, but long-neglected, part of treating your food obsession. On this walk, you will meet and greet a lost essential self. This meeting is absolutely necessary to achieve *permanent* weight loss. Whether you need professional mentors, friendly support, or travels to distant lands, stay awake and pay attention.

How will you know when you meet your Buddha on the road? What does your spiritual self look like? What does "spiritual" mean? Could a gutsy, tough, and headstrong New Yorker be spiritual? Or does being spiritual mean giving up to become a dishrag? Can you just wave a white flag and be zapped thin? How would a person know if he or she actually surrendered?

You'll know you've surrendered when you notice the following:

Symptoms of a Spiritual Awakening

1. Acting spontaneously without past fears.

2. Loss of interest in judging people.

3. A tendency to let things happen, giving up control.

4. Praying toward heaven while rowing toward shore.

5. Loss of interest in conflict.

6. Appreciating the body's function rather than its form.

7. Loss of the ability to worry.

8. Frequent reminders that "if you spot it, you got it."

9. Understanding that "they do it not *to* you, but *for* them."

10. Trusting of your instincts, others, and nature.

11. Attitude of gratitude and abundance.

12. Personal acceptance, warts and all.

"If you are willing

to serenely bear the trial

of being displeasing to yourself,

then you will be for all

a pleasant place of shelter."

ST. THÉRÈSE OF LISIEUX

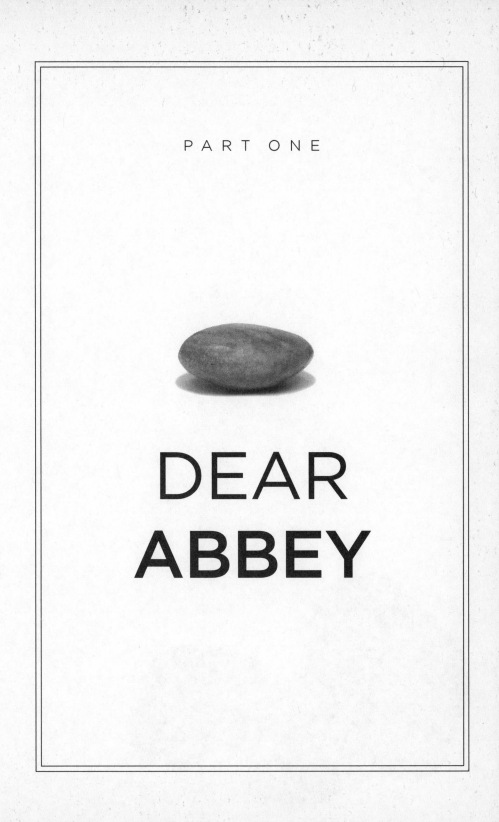

PART ONE

DEAR
ABBEY

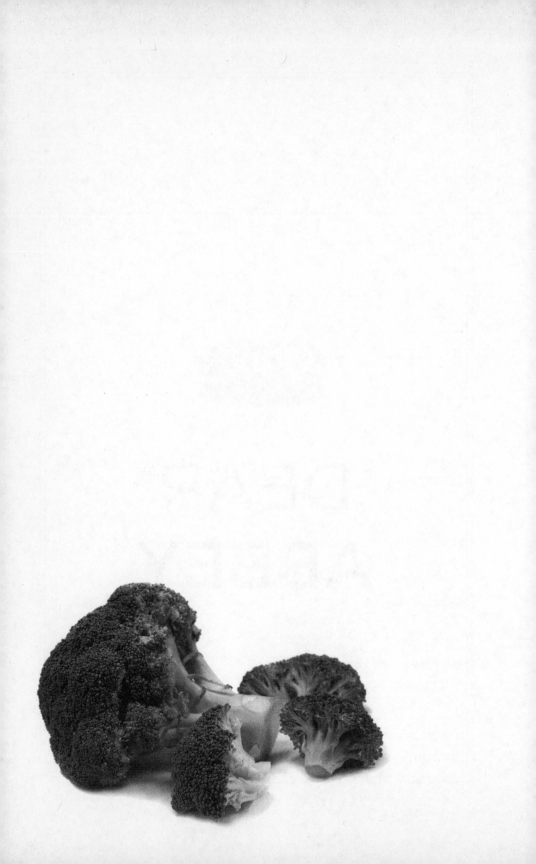

ONE
Hit a Wall

1983

Jewish girls don't bow, kneel, or genuflect . . . except in bed, of course.

So what's a nice Jewish girl like me doing in a place like this?

A Buddhist monastery, no less.

Something I ate?

No, I guess it's what I don't *eat that's brought me to this.*

When I pass through this chicken-wire gate, I, who make my living talking, will join others who are committed to total silence. I have been auditioning to enter this place for months.

Surrounded by pine-scented woods facing a large volcanic mountain, I listen to the stark alpine quiet that will be my home and wonder why I'm here.

At age ten I weighed exactly what I do now as a mature, premenopausal woman. Just before my tenth birthday, after dieting away thirty pounds, I went to a local malt shop to flirt. I wore a tight maroon skirt with wide black belt, bobby socks, and saddle oxfords. I was allowed to sip a milk shake, sucking the glass dry, as long as I didn't have sex. In those days, sex was forbidden but chocolate indulged. Today it's the other way around.

From then on, despite TOFU (The Occasional Foul-Up), I white-knuckled it most of the time, and then repeatedly picked myself up from those slips and got back on the horse. Though now seventy pounds lighter than my top weight, with approaching menopause, I am slowly regaining some weight.

That's how I ended up in a small plane headed toward the Oregon border and Shasta Abbey with Yves, my lover and business partner, flying us in his beloved Bellanca Viking, a single–engine, wooden-winged aircraft named Lucy.

I'm always scared flying in Lucy as she takes us halfway across the country to my various lecture gigs and TV appearances. Sometimes we fly above 12,000 feet, requiring oxygen masks. One time, as we waited on the ground in Texas, Yves turned to me, white-faced, and said, "The wind shears and thunderstorms are too heavy. You go on ahead with a commercial jet while Lucy and I wait out the storm." Another time while in Denver, we had to do numerous fly-bys to ascertain from the tower, "Yes, your landing gear is locked in the down position. Over." Quite honestly, I figured that since we have to land again anyway, we should keep the gear down for the duration. Instead, we stayed over to get it fixed. What do I know about planes?

Anticipating more such surprises to delay my flight to Shasta Abbey, I bury myself in magazines and pistachio nuts. After a rather uneventful trip, Yves settles into a motel and we sit down to share a late supper. Consequently, I arrive at the abbey behind schedule.

While awaiting admittance through the chicken-wire gate, I ponder all it took to get me here.

I try to remember why or how I've come to this place. I know I fought really hard to get here. But why?

I didn't even have a clue how I'd received the summer workshop brochure from the abbey.

Even though I am thin and successful, I am increasingly restless and bored. I know I need deeper connections. I'm in that state of perpetual longing, like when I leave that last bite of chocolate cake.

How often does that happen?

Despite decades of professional accolades, thousands applauding my message, asking for my autograph or photo, I never felt deserving of what came my way. I felt like an imposter, a rotten, bad seed. That fueled my hurried, workaholic overscheduling. It had everything to do with my overeating as well.

I never relaxed enough to enjoy the journey. I never surrendered to a spiritual way of life. I didn't look or act like any of the people who appeared to be spiritual. They seemed calmer. They believed in God or believed in some kind of a universal oneness: "We're all connected." I didn't get any of it. I didn't buy into the God concept and relished being in charge of my life and the lives of others, even if I was a bad apple. I'm sure that rotten-to-the-core feeling caused my periodic returns to bouts of compulsive eating; my self-destruct button was still intact.

So, anticipating a chance to get away from the daily emergencies at my HOPE House treatment center, I'd called Shasta Abbey. I'd learned I enjoyed brief forays into the spiritual life, but I really didn't crave *total* transformation. I wanted to lose weight, change a little maybe, but keep my winning personality.

Half a year earlier, on my first inquiry over the phone, I listen while on hold, trying to organize a monastery stay, when my reverie is broken with "How did you hear about us?"

Reverend Kincaid questions me softly as I plot my course from spiritual neophyte to awakened Zen master. *This monk has a noticeable New York accent.* I sense his hesitancy.

"What brings you to call us? What is your experience with Buddhism or meditation?"

"Well, Reverend Kincaid, sir, I became a therapist to figure out why I ate. Some of the things I learned were so depressing that I *ate over them*. Though I believe I am a gifted therapist, I find my relationship with food is best when I stop trying to figure it out and instead consult my stillness within. I eventually found that spiritual principles helped me more than intellect.

"So I found your brochure and I am drawn to this 'Life of the Buddha' retreat. It says here in your brochure, 'The Buddha lived a daily life facing unjust criticism, envy, mistakes in judgment, and exhaustion.' Well, both the Buddha and I have similar struggles," I pompously state.

"But why Buddhism?" "Well, I've been following Baba Ram Dass since the 1960s."

I wonder if Reverend Kincaid knows that Ram Dass is a spiritual leader who dropped acid with Timothy Leary, gave up his name of Richard Alpert along with the status of Harvard professor, and dedicated himself to traveling to and from India while transforming America's youth.

"Ram Dass taught us to let go and consult our own souls for direction, but he also advised us to live spiritual principles in everyday life. Just because we commune with the Gods and Goddesses is no reason not to know our postal zip code."

Pleading into the receiver, I beg Reverend Kincaid to let me sign up. "I know it's a three-week workshop, but I can only get away for the last week. I'm sure I can catch up."

As usual, I wanted special permission, offering, "My case is different. I deserve special consideration."

Reverend Kincaid responds kindly, "I appreciate your interest, but I suggest you first attend an introductory workshop. Or perhaps you would benefit more from the beginner's week-long retreat that focuses on basic teachings and practice."

Doesn't he understand? I can't get away so easily. I'm booked!

"It will be too much for you to plop into the third week of training with no background. Others already there will be way ahead of you and it will be difficult for you to catch up."

He concludes with "Let me send you our informational packet for you to consider what's in store."

When the "Guest Information" packet arrives, I read it over hurriedly along with the "Introduction to Soto Zen" and immediately call again. In my zeal, I dismiss the brochure's caution that in the beginning attendees "experience some difficulty with specific aspects of training."

Not applicable to me.

As he answers my call, Reverend Kincaid returns once again to his initial query about how I'd received the brochure. "We just don't have an extensive mailing list," he sniffs.

I know he senses the absence of incense in my voice.

"Have you ever meditated before?" he grills.

Knowing my answer may now disqualify me, I quickly lie, "I have meditated intermittently, and have a deep spiritual consciousness." I hope he won't ask me what that means. I can't honestly say.

My quick lie sounds good to me. My "meditations" are often brief interludes when I space out watching cars pass by my window or while I'm looking out at waves breaking on the shore.

More often, however, I spend meditation time in "monkey mind," busy with planning, manipulating, decorating, investigating, arguing, justifying, or daydreaming. No matter how brief or unfocused these episodes, I am sure they qualify me to be on some imagined meditation checklist. Determined as I am to get accepted, my further entreaties to Reverend Kincaid mimic the best college fullback's melodrama:

"Let me at 'em, coach."

"Just this once for the Buddha!"

Challenged by my desire to get *what* I want *when* I want it, I set out to convince this monk I can make the grade.

That's the only week I have free.

Doesn't he realize what an important and busy person I am? My schedule is booked well over a year in advance. I appear regularly on all the national shows. As a recognized expert in counseling addicted families, I'm giving lectures and seminars throughout the country training medical professionals to treat bulimia, anorexia, and compulsive eating. Surely I needn't beg to attend a workshop. And I have to work there, too? "Jewish psychologist begs Buddhist monk for chance to sell self into monastic slavery." What is definitely wrong with this picture?

He should realize how lucky they are to have me. Why, if I like the place, I'll recommend it to others. I could greatly improve their business.

I continue auditioning for this Queens-sounding monk whose title is "Guestmaster of the Abbey." Respectfully, I work to enhance my cause, explaining my importance—a pioneering legend in my own mind.

"Reverend, sir, I created the nation's first eating disorders unit. I'm author of the bestseller *Fat Is a Family Affair.* I direct thriving clinics in three states, and countless imitations are springing up all over the US. I teach people how their obsessions for excess food are really part of a larger hunger for a spiritual connection."

I'm spiritual, by God!

I try impressing him with psychobabble. "You see, I know a lot about these matters. As a matter of fact, Carl Jung explained to Bill W, one of the cofounders of Alcoholics Anonymous, that understanding psychological causalities would not relieve spiritual hunger the way going inward and living spiritually could. He said addicts suffer 'a hole in the soul.' And that's why I want to develop more spiritual practice." I know he'll agree to accept me; surely I have enough background to come in during the third week and catch up.

Instead of offering me the coveted "yes" right away, Reverend Kincaid responds softly, "I'll send you further explanation of our practice and see if you feel you could benefit from it."

Duly challenged, I set out to make it to the abbey. I operate from some inexplicable longing to fully immerse myself in meditation and contemplation (but only for one week). Why I choose this particular format is still a mystery. Why would an army brat who'd traveled the world long to be on a mountaintop in Northern California? Why here? Why now?

Reverend Kincaid grills me further. "You'll notice that we have job assignments, known as *samu,* working meditation."

"Oh, I know about such things. I've been training addiction counselors for decades, and I am a consultant to numerous treatment centers. At HOPE House, my own residential treatment center, new arrivals are given job responsibilities and are expected to produce and live up to their commitments. We've found that low self-esteem is quickly healed with successful completion of assigned tasks. I understand hard work. I won't 'wimp out' on you. For now, I just want a chance to get away. I want to step down from my guru role and get out of the obligations of management. I don't want to be the one with the answers. I want to be a newcomer—little know-nothing *shmegegge*."

Assuring the Guestmaster of my willingness to meditate, my understanding of the concept of work as a meditative, therapeutic necessity, I still have to convince him I am spiritual.

"I've spent many years working with self-help groups; studied Gestalt and family therapy, psychodrama, psychosynthesis, transpersonal psychology, and est. I've made three sojourns throughout Southeast Asia and India, and I've even led retreats at Omega and Esalen institutes."

Finally, Reverend Kincaid agrees to admit me to the third week of training without further objection. Little can he know how I will contrast with the other trainees at the abbey.

Okay, so I have hot pink nails and bright maroon hair. Cellophane hair colors are in. And, despite my appetite for spirituality, I still adore high fashion, glitzy bling-bling earrings, tight jeans, and a smattering of street talk. Why should I worry? Don't monks believe in acceptance?

Winning the audition and finally getting my way, I forge ahead obsessively. After rearranging my schedule to get my hair permed before leaving, I begin worrying about my nails, so I pack rubber gloves. After all, my nail job costs almost as much as the entire week at this monastery.

In addition to my computer, CDs, and "nonscented" toiletries (as instructed), I separate out reading materials for the plane trips hither and yon. Abbey rules suggest reading only Buddhist literature while in residence. I have a healthy cache of magazines like *Parade, Family Circle,* and *Drama-Logue* for some escapist diversion going in and out of serenity city.

Thinking I'm getting away with something, I subvert abbey rules for moderate dress and no perfume or makeup by defiantly packing sexy lace underwear. I am still insisting on having it my way, making my decisions about what rules I will or will not follow.

I can't go to the abbey without some trappings from home, so I pack CDs of old-time blues ladies wailing sexy songs. Despite whatever meditative brainwashing these monks might shower on me by day, I intend to retreat to my room at night under the canopy of raunchy blues to strut and grind the night away.

Of course, as ever, my major problem is "What to wear?" Abbey literature is quite specific. Meditation sessions of up to three hours require a long, full skirt of subdued color, so as not to disturb the meditative practice of others.

Their brochure suggests bringing various weights of blouses and sweaters, considering the highly unpredictable weather on the mountain. "Baggy jeans for work detail" are no problem, as are sleeping bag, toiletries, proper shoes, and heavy jacket. But no matter what I draw out of my closet, each item shines in bright neon compared to the quiet subtlety of Kincaid's voice. My bright pinks, golds, oranges, and whites have been carefully selected to complement a perennial Southern California tan. "Subtle" is a word foreign to the "casual, nonprofessional" section of my closet.

I make one especially frantic call quizzing Kincaid. "Are flowers okay?"

That same lilting, slightly East Coast voice responds, "Why of course, as long as it's not something terribly loud and garish, such as Hawaiian prints."

Okay, back on the hanger goes my favorite purple, yellow, green, and gold Anne Pinkerton jungle print.

Doesn't he understand that I live a bicoastal life, mostly in Manhattan Beach, California? We dress to play, not to pray.

I finally give in and buy a khaki-green full skirt, which matches a khaki sweater, and then I throw in my beige Western cowgirl skirt. I know that without the boots I'll pass for spiritual rather than honky-tonk—cheap and superficial.

Prepared for all options, I'm quite proud when I manage to cram all into two "small" valises and a sleeping bag pouch. Only on the plane trip up do I reread the brochure to find "only one suitcase" is allowed. Dead in the water, I resolve to make it through a less-than-perfect week.

And that's how I finally arrive—late and inappropriate.

Ambling toward the chain-link fence is Reverend Kincaid, all towering six feet of him. I'm surprised. *Aren't monks supposed to be shorter and more gnomelike?* His long brown robes and cape rustle toward me. *His head looks funny.* Shaved, but hair is partially grown out. I'll later learn he's preparing for a "home visit." His large, round, brown eyes look away as he offers no gratuitous welcoming smile or greeting.

Doesn't he know who I am?

He swings aside the rickety gate, dragging its rollers just enough for me and my bags to get through. This light, wobbly gate, easily moved to allow quick entry, doesn't at all foretell the heaviness I'll push against later. This man, whose gentle voice so scared me on the phone and who quietly, carefully, and repeatedly warned me, finally appears in the flesh. I'm so excited.

He's not.

He just seems focused on getting the job done. *Boy, at my centers we're a lot friendlier.* As trained treatment professionals, understanding how frightened incoming patients might be, we make sure they know they are entering a place where we *know* them, *see* them, and will take good *care* of them. Reverend Kincaid signals none of that. Instead of offering any reassuring politeness, he moves as if our mission is already written—that I am supposed to be there and that we are performing functions already prescribed and expected. There is no need to comment. He never really makes eye contact with me, but rather eyes my luggage. Helping me drag the two heavy valises down to the arrivals cottage, he never reminds me that the brochure recommends "bring only one bag."

After sitting down for my formal introduction in the arrivals cottage, he asks, "Do you have any questions?"

I beam from the edge of my seat in all exuberance, shrugging. "No, not really. I'm so happy and excited to be here."

Inhaling deeply, he reminds me that abbey rules prohibit makeup or perfumes.

I apologize. "Oh, this is all leftovers from the trip up here. I'll be clean as a whistle as soon as I get to my room. I'll change clothes, kick off the cowboy boots, and wash off all the perfume."

His voice seems to boom gently, but ominously, "Yooooouuuuuu hhhhhaaaaaaaaaaaavvve nooooooooooo rrrooooooooooommmmmm."

I let it pass.

He turns me over to Reverend Muldoon, whose head sprouts strawberry-blonde stubble. As she gives me a tour of the grounds, she explains *gassho,* which is a formal bowing with hands folded firmly and flatly, thumbs together toward chest, fingers heavenward. "You will practice *gassho* respectfully, acknowledging those people, places, or things appreciated."

She doesn't really know who I am. I've been around spirituality camps for years. I know gassho. *I've been observing Dürer's famous "praying hands" plastered just above the Serenity Prayer on greeting cards or dangling as lockets and charms around the necks of countless twelve-step members.*

She demonstrates a few of the required and suggested opportunities for bowing. "You will bow entering and leaving certain buildings. Eating halls and bathrooms are cause for special bowing in gratitude. Without question, you will bow entering and leaving the temple, and definitely when facing the large Buddha statue, along with a number of other shrines around the property. Just follow the practice of other trainees. They will model for you correct behaviors. Buddhism is about being respectful to every living thing and trying to do no harm.

"In our processions, the lead monk carries a walking stick topped by a small bell that tinkles slightly. This is to warn bugs on the path to move aside, so as not to be trampled by the oncoming slippers.

"Everyone works and has purpose here at the abbey. Even little children are assigned the job of sweeping bugs gently off the path. If any bug meets an inadvertent early demise, funeral services are performed immediately."

Geez, I wonder if she knows I massacred a lowly cockroach last week.

"As part of being respectful to all living things, our living code, called "precepts," recommends that we remain mindful and pay attention and have consciousness about what we do and what effects our actions create. At the same time, we strive to proceed in an unselfconscious manner, losing ourselves in action. Life must be lived as a meditation. In meditation, we are to neither hold on nor push away, taking a gentle, neutral stance. We also try to behave in a way that will not embarrass or offend ourselves or others.

"For example," she continues, now facing me with direct eye contact, "Your blouse, although quite acceptable in your world, might be a bit low-cut for our standards here at the abbey. We do not call attention to anything that would disturb the meditative practice of others."

Boy, her smock seems awfully lightweight, and when she stands in the sun it looks like she wears no underwear.

Instead of casting these pearls, I quickly assure her, "As soon as I get to my room, I'll change into something more appropriate."

"Yooooouuuuuu hhhhhaaaaaaaaaaavvve noooooooooo rrrooooooooommmmm," she says, echoing Kincaid, as she leads me back to the guest cottage where bags are neatly stowed.

This "no room" line has a menacing echo to it.

Still, I let it pass.

As we arrive at the guest cottage, Reverend Muldoon further explains, "Your bags will be stored in the luggage room for the duration of your stay. You will have personal space in the bathhouse to store any articles of immediate need."

She shows me my personal space: three shelves, each measuring four inches by six inches.

My name is emblazoned smartly above each cigar-box- sized cubicle. It is immediately and abundantly clear that I'll be making numerous treks from luggage room to bathhouse. *But where will I sleep?*

No time for that.

Being such a novice, I'm taken to Reverend Penelope for meditation instruction.

"You mean you are brand-new and you've come in the middle of a three-week retreat?" she asks, intimating it might be difficult for me.

"Well, this was the only time I could get away," I answer importantly, "and I wanted to fully immerse myself in the experience. I work in the field."

By now I seem to be embarrassing myself with every word. My "field" might just be a pasture where I'm already knee-deep in cow pies.

Glad she doesn't ask for an explanation, I continue jabbering. "I feel like a sponge soaking everything up for the first time."

"Ah, we call that 'beginner's mind,' which makes you quite receptive, and you will learn a great deal."

I'm now bug-eyed as Penelope proceeds with her lessons. In some twelve-step programs, "beginner's mind" is referred to as "newcomer eyes." They resemble a deer caught in headlights. Lending me a meditation skirt, as there is no time to unpack my own, she shows me the suggested meditative practice. "The round pillow, *zafu,* is often used to facilitate sitting in the lotus position: legs folded upon each other so that one's spine is fully supported and free for consciousness to enter or leave the body. Some find the meditation stool easier and others sit straight on an elevated backless bench."

She demonstrates all options.

"Which is best?" I inquire.

"None is best. It's just important to find what works for you."

I figure, *Anyone worth her salt should pull a lotus.*

Determined to become expert with my first attempt at meditation, I go for the *zafu*. Penelope asks me to get in position so she can help me find the proper breathing and muscle tone. I quickly hop onto the *zafu*, but find that my folded knees don't touch the floor.

Penelope, ever so kindly, suggests that I try using the stool. "It allows leaning back in a kneeling position." *More Christian than Buddhist*, I think. I decide to shut up and listen as I surmise I've already flunked Meditation 101.

I absentmindedly accept the stool and don't even wait to notice how it feels. *I just know I won't resort to any elevated cop-out. I want total immersion. No matter what coach, I won't be benched.*

"You'll have time after dinner to unpack a few things," Reverend Penelope instructs as she directs me to the temple where meditation is due to begin.

Now my head races, recalling explanations in the Guest Information brochure.

Wow, a lot of each day is spent staring blankly at a bare white wall. I might have bitten off more than even a well-heeled compulsive overeater can swallow.

Panic arises as I realize I might find difficulty sitting for a full week of *zazen* meditation. My mind races quickly, remembering the schedule Kincaid sent. There will be six meditation sessions each day separated by three different work assignments, one or two classes, and two quiet reading periods. There will also be two brief chances to rest—to be used for showering, gift shop, or phone calls.

Each different activity will require costume changes from work to eating, to class, or to meditation clothes. I'll be doing heavy trekking to the storage room to accommodate all the required costume changes. This does not even account for weather changes. Abbey climate in June necessitates more wardrobe changes than an elaborate Broadway musical.

What have I gotten myself into?

No time to consider such trifles now. I must hurry up to relax into meditation.

As I hightail it up to the temple, the cloisters are filled with monks scurrying to new locations. I have no idea how difficult navigation will be as I walk up the incline for each activity and costume change.

No dawdling on the path is allowed. Silence is preferred, with necessary conversation kept at whisper pitch. Leisurely strolls filled with polite chitchat about weather, meals, and such do not exist. Abbey time is to be spent going within and staying centered.

If you pass another on the path, you can offer *gassho* to acknowledge contact. That's it. No talking, smiling, indicating, or performing. Just hello and goodbye.

A vague sense of loneliness and fear begins to creep up within me. No time to think of that now. I bravely embrace Scarlett O'Hara's philosophy of thinking about "it" tomorrow.

However, my tomorrow arrives quite ahead of schedule.

I hurry to the temple, bowing at two shrines on the way. Depositing my cowboy boots alongside a neatly placed lineup of healthy hiking sandals, I swing open the heavy iron-handled door to enter the temple.

Inside it is cold, dark, and damp compared to the bright, airy sunlight I've just run through. I can barely make out the other trainees seated along the periphery. All are lined up and seated, facing white walls. Reverend Kincaid had advised, "When in doubt, just follow the practice of others and you'll catch on." A tall, lanky, bearded man in a white skirt directly ahead of me bows to the room, bows to the fifty-foot Buddha statue, and then quietly walks to the other side of the temple.

I do the same.

He then bows to his wall space, turns and bows again to the Buddha, and seats himself on his cushion facing the wall. As my movie-theater blindness clears, I see more people and Penelope's meditation instructions call out from the back of my head. Imagining a square dance caller's bark, I'm pushed to similarly bow low, "honor my corner, honor my partner," and settle in on my stool. A gong is sounded and a monk announces, "Meditation."

We now sit for thirty minutes. I go at this with a Western Protestant work ethic, resolving to muddle through no matter what. Within ten minutes a tingling numbness races past my knees up to my thighs. I'd heard that *zazen* meditation could become uncomfortable, but one should focus away from the pain and on one's breathing and not allow physical pettiness to keep you from Nirvana.

The numbness in my limbs is actually a welcome relief compared to the excruciating, hatchet-like attack in the center of my forehead—certainly a mega-migraine. Since it's after 4:00 p.m., this is probably the result of major caffeine withdrawal. "Going to God no matter what," I become "one with," although I'm not sure with what. I try to settle in and even out my breathing.

Hardly noticing the time pass, I hear a deeper brass gong and then a monk's soft voice announce, "Walking meditation." I note tremendous rustling as all stooped bodies become erect and begin a slow walk. As I kick back my stool, my legs shoot forward like matchsticks. No matter how much my Western mind urges me to get upright, I roll over onto the sides of my feet and buckle under. Undaunted, I push and work my way up like a grasshopper, immediately crumbling onto the rug. Feeling no sensation from my hip socket down, I have no fear of amputation, just embarrassment that I can't get up from the floor.

Reverend Penelope's voice whispers close to my ear, "Are you having trouble, Judi?"

"Is the pope Catholic?" I want to scream at her naked earlobe. I nod instead.

"I think you'd better try the bench. Come, I'll find you a place." She holds my elbow and we waddle over together. Sitting through the second stage with "old" ladies on the bench, demoralized at my "failure," I don't even notice how many others chose this more practical perch.

When meditation ends, I finally find the answer to that mysterious "nooooooo rrroooooommmmmm."

Reverend Kincaid enters the darkened hall, flipping on the lights to alert our squinting eyes and announcing melodiously, as he's no doubt done for the previous two weeks of the retreat, "We will now prepare a chamber for sleeping."

All of the retreat trainees huddled below the Buddha statue know their assigned roles (except for me) as they bow to the Buddha, bow to the door, and then race down a ramp to a storeroom filled with sleeping mats and room divider screens. They scurry like squirrels, each grabbing a screen and bowing to Buddha on the way back in.

The screens are set up to create a division between the male and female sides of the hall. All carry in futon mats, each knowing which one is his or her own. After placing sleeping bags atop these futons, they rush quickly out to the "conversational tea." We are scheduled to be there to make small talk with selected monks. But I'm having none of it.

Observing this human anthill hurriedly moving large objects, I stare straight ahead, totally transfixed. My breathing is shallow and I'm clueless as to how to proceed. Reverend Kincaid stirs me out of my stupor. "Judi, would you like to choose a mat?"

I rush to comply as neither of us notices the large tears swimming along the rims of my eyes. Overcome with a sick feeling of flight like a threatened animal in the wild, I want to relieve myself and gallop off.

I'm expected to sleep in this large hall with all these other trainees? No privacy? No walkman? No rrrrrrooooommmmm!

I've found my room, but hit the wall.

TWO
Lean into It

Too much is just too much.

I must have a room. I like my comfort. I need privacy. I have music to play.

I begin planning my escape.

I've done all they said. I've willingly crushed my legs under the stool, pushed leaden limbs erect, and now dragged a futon to the last empty female space in the shrine. I'm obediently accepting whatever is put in front of me, but enough is enough. I can't take any more. Without a chance for privacy, I can't last.

In a daze, I spread out my mat and push myself to the next scheduled activity: the monk's "conversational tea."

I don't bow one *gassho* at any shrine on the way, and then, in a tearful trance, I enter the recreation room where Reverend Paul leads the tea party. He's telling cute stories while old-timer trainees giggle and sip. They're serving newly picked cherries. I scoop myself a bowl and begin popping them absentmindedly, spitting pits and stems back into the same bowl. Tears now unashamedly roll down my cheeks.

I have to leave.

I just can't take one more minute of this place.

I run out, and, despite the Buddhist exhortation against wasting food, I toss my cherries, pits, stems, and all into the nearest trash bin. After racing back to the luggage room to get quarters, I leap cloisters hurriedly to reach the public phone booth.

I call Yves's motel. "You've got to get me out of this place. I can't take it. I don't belong here. Kincaid was right; I shouldn't have started midstream." I sob and gulp.

Yves, in his deep, mellow, radio-announcer tones, coos, "Oh, poor baby. You're really having a hard time, aren't you?" Despite the fact I'd initially fallen in love with his gentle, soothing voice, I have no time for that comfort crap now. (We'd had a phone romance for three months before we actually met. He told me then, "I give great phone.")

Phone, shmone; like E.T., *I want home.*

Keeping up my gently oozing sobs, I can't think of anything else to say.

Yves asks, "Have you talked with anyone there about this?"

"No," I whine, and the rest tumbles out quickly. "I don't know what to say. They're all very nice, friendly, happy folks. I can't take the bowing. I don't have a room. We sleep on the floor. There's no free time. I'll never get to use my computer or hear my music. I can't sit on a stool. My legs are giving out. I don't know how to meditate. I don't know why I'm doing this. I just can't take the bowing. We have to bow at everything!"

"I think you're feeling really lonely," he soothes in his best silver-tongued-devil voice. "Why don't you talk to someone there first, and then if you want I'll definitely come and get you. Could you hold out 'til morning? I'll come for you in the morning if you decide to leave."

"Okay," I sob. "I'll talk with them. They're having tea now. I can't interrupt the tea. I'll go back and listen. I just don't understand what I'm doing here. Is this for the benefit of my patients or what? I don't need to be doing this. Let me read a book. I'm not a Buddhist."

"Jude, it's about control. They're taking away your power. You're in a scary new place where no one knows what an important person you are. You aren't in the power position. You don't have all your usual trappings of contentment. There's no podium or image to hide behind. No one wants to hear your words of wisdom or see your winning personality. You're just there for you to go inward and get to know yourself. If you can stick it out, you'll probably get a lot from it. Remember, you said you weren't *attached* to your lifestyle, your possessions, your position, or your things. You tell people in your lectures that you can walk away from anything whenever you want. Now is the time for you to walk your talk."

Damn. I know he's right.

I just sob harder.

"Honey, you sound just like one of our patients," he says with a loving smile in his tone.

I shriek, "I know that. I *know* that. I understand exactly what I'm doing and what's going on. I see it all clearly, and I don't care. I don't care, shmare, wear, bear! WHATEVER! I just want OUT."

I regret every day I've ever shared with him those family therapy principles about "release with love," or letting people "work their own side of the street," or "no pain, no gain," or any of that crap.

I growl, "Call you back in the morning," and then slam down the receiver.

Crying all the way back to tea, I reenter with crazed, crimson eyes, glaring at all their contented, tea-soaked grins. When his speech ends, I approach Reverend Paul and quiver. "Can I talk with you?"

Smiling quietly, he asks, "About what?"

That's it. The floodgates burst as I now sob uncontrollably. Ushering me gently out the door, he sits us down on the kitchen stairs.

I begin blankly. "I have to leave, and I thought I should talk to someone first," I boohoo, getting out all my frustrations and fears.

"Everyone's great here. It's a great place. It could be a great time, but I just have to go. I just can't stop crying."

"There's nothing wrong with crying," he answers, staring quietly straight ahead.

I boohoo more.

After a minute, he gently faces me dead-on. "This place makes you come up against yourself. It's quite frightening. You can't run or hide anywhere. It makes one go inward, deeper, and closer to the real Self."

How the hell does this guy know about me? I'm not afraid. I just have a lot of things to do and don't really see the value of wasting a week with this. I just don't have enough motivation or desperation to stick it out. After all, my patients want freedom from food obsessions. They're suffering and seeking relief. I've already done that. I'm doing quite well, thank you very much. I don't want or need anything. I surely don't need this. I must be on some stupid kick to investigate alternative lifestyles. This is an intellectual mission of mercy to benefit my staff and patients. I've made a mistake. I don't need to put myself through this.

"I love my life," I scream at his bald head. "I don't want to be a monk."

He slowly turns toward me again and gently responds to my panic. He breathes, and then pauses before speaking. "No one here would ask you to give up anything about your life. Principles you learn here can be carried back to your world, or not. It is true, however, that once you see and experience the truth, it burns like a fire within and you can't pretend you haven't seen or known it. I've obviously made my choice about things."

His shaved head bears witness.

"Do you think you could make it through until tomorrow, or should I get Reverend Kincaid? We can get someone to drive you into town right now if that's what you'd like."

Secured by some returning sense of power, and also aware I've promised Yves I'll wait until morning, I assure him I can make it through the night. He comforts me further with "Perhaps a good night's sleep will make things clearer."

Before reaching the women's bathhouse, I'm approached by Reverend Kincaid.

Who ratted on me?

He begins gently with "Let's sit here by the fountain and talk." I make my way over and sit down to sob some more.

"I told you it might be hard to jump in midstream," he reminds me.

"I know, I know," I screech. "You were right, you were right. I shouldn't have come. It's the bowing. I can't take the bowing. I don't want to be a monk. I just wanted to study how Buddha's principles work in the world."

"I'd better go home and read more. I really thought I'd have some space and time to think. I'm just a dilettante. I never should have come. You're all very nice. Everyone's been wonderful. I just can't stop crying. I can't figure out the bowing. I've got to go."

Reverend Kincaid showers me with the same gentleness shown by Reverend Paul. With no attempt to convince me of anything and with no condescension, he replies, "Rituals, such as bowing, are here to develop a certain orientation or practice, but they are really reminders of deeper meanings. The principles of gratitude, love, and service that you practice by bowing can be incorporated back to life outside of here. You are experiencing a loss of your normal structures and it is forcing you to move to other levels with which you have not yet been acquainted. We provide you with enough structure so that you can feel free to move to deeper levels without worry. We are freeing your mind of some decisions so you may focus on others and so that you can let go."

Could it be that this dear man actually knows how much of my life is spent organizing my closet, scheduling appointments, and devising new treatment plans for patients? If my body and soul were not occupied with such diversions, what would I think about?

Oh, I get it. This is about not thinking at all.

What will my head do all day long? Even if that dilemma was solved, what about my room? Doesn't he know my zodiac sign is Cancer? We need to nest.

"But despite all my best intentions, I can't even do this stuff!" I seem to be screeching into yet another naked ear socket. "I couldn't even meditate on a stool. I had to be benched."

He stares directly ahead, not looking at me, just like Reverend Paul, and, with a slight smile, answers, "I use the bench."

Yet another image shattered!

Eyes bugged in amazement, I wonder, *How could the "Guestmaster of the Abbey" not sit in lotus position on a pillow?*

Don't these people know anything about leadership qualities and motivational techniques? I'm totally giving up on expecting any professionalism.

He interrupts my head's rant. "You seem extremely wound up right now. Perhaps a good night's sleep will help you sort things out."

Thanking him profusely for all his kindness, I apologize for my panic and tears.

"Why don't you take time out of the morning cleanup schedule to make your decision? I'll relieve you of any work detail so you can meditate more, make necessary phone calls, and then either fully participate or jump ship."

"Sure. Thanks again for everything." Smiling a sweet goodnight, I leave him to tiptoe into the temple past inert forms already cuddled into their sleeping bags. I crawl into mine and begin a quiet sob. Torn and disappointed and totally confused, I finally fall asleep. The Reverend and I both know I'll be leaving in the morning.

But morning finds me still unresolved. I certainly feel increased compassion for those poor patients who'd come to HOPE House for treatment. Many had left their secure homes in the Midwest or even from faraway Spain, Sweden, or Hong Kong to come to the Mecca of eating disorder treatment, HOPE House, Hollywood. I empathized with their disappointment and fear of facing themselves and their lives. I understand now exactly what was going on. After all, I am a therapist. Even so, I still want out.

I remember there were those few crazed patients who ran off in the middle of the night, then called us next day from hotel rooms, pleading to return to treatment. I now clearly understand what they meant when they cried, "I don't know why I ran. I just had to get away." The open-door policies of Shasta Abbey and HOPE House are both a blessing and an equal curse. I'd welcome more restrictions to limit my choices.

I'd like to be bound and gagged to enlightenment, please.

When morning comes, I hurry out to the north woods of the abbey, hoping to question myself one more time to finally come to some decision. Each minute I vacillate. One second I have firm resolve to stick it out, trusting in possible future benefits; then, in an instant, I reverse course, clamoring, "Who needs this? This is a real waste of time. This place works for some displaced sixties hippies, but what do their choices have to do with my life?"

Reverend Kincaid meets up with me on the path. I look in his eyes and start to cry. "I want to stay. I just don't think I *can*."

He answers simply, "Anyone can. You first need to resolve if you want to. If you want to, then you can. Just do your best. That's all anyone can do. In Buddhism we say, 'begin at once and do your best.'"

Such clarity.

His simple statement bores softly into my heart as the pine needles rustle a bit in the still morning calm. My crying stops as I face him and myself.

Of course, what else could I do but my best? What else can anyone do? Who cares, anyway? Who's watching or evaluating? Judge Judi's the only judge in the room. No one else notices. No one cares. This experience is totally for me.

But I just want my own room, a little privacy, a little chance to think or write alone. I want, I want, I want . . . a chance to hear Bessie Smith's bluesy wail.

Ladies who sing the blues know how to fight. So do I. Why don't these monks try to fight to convince me to stay? Battling is easy. I already have good arguments: Didn't they see how ill-prepared I was and how it was all their fault? I know whom to blame. If they would have just told me about all this bowing.

My self-justification looms up with "It's their disorganization that worries me."

I want control. I want to handle it. I want a guarantee. I want ice cream. I want to know that I won't change and this place will not affect me. I want. I want. I want.

I recall how much I'd looked forward to this week with such enthusiasm and excitement.

Couldn't I recapture some of that spirit of adventure, go ahead and accept their structure, but not necessarily lose myself? Can't I hold on to some of my discerning eye and maintain perspective? Why not make the most of it? I can stop feeling so responsible, blaming myself for "choosing" to be here. Hell, I don't even know how or why I'd received the brochure.

As the initial wave of fear begins to subside, I feel such love from these monks. I'm clearly not afraid of them or their rules; I'm afraid of me. What might I learn about me? I have met the enemy and she looks like *me.*

With no one to fight, the answer comes slowly but clearly.

I face Reverend Kincaid with no tears, just a straight stare of confidence and a determined tone in my voice. "I'll stay."

I'll apply the same principle that has kept my food in order for many years: "One day at a time." If it becomes unbearable, I'll just pack up and move on. Just for today, I can take it. I am willing to stay for one full day.

Countdown begins . . .

THREE
One Day at a Time

My first morning. I arrive early at the bare-bones dining hall. All trainees line up alongside steel tables surrounded by folding chairs. A soft bell sounds and pandemonium ensues. Chairs screeching along the flagstone floor disturb my early-morning stupor. Once we're all seated, the din subsides as bowls are passed with silent *gasshos.*

Breakfast is cardboard.

Tears keep streaming down my cheeks while I chew laboriously, staring blankly. *Who cares about food at a time like this?* Meals at the abbey are eaten in silence with accompanying rituals and prayers, and, of course, bows. In this environment of love and honesty, openness and respect, all I can do is cry.

Stop crying.

Finish up.

Bow to your plate.

Scrape leftovers into the "compost" can.

Bow to it.

Scurry over to the "job assignments" monk.

Bow to him.

He finds my name on his clipboard and says, "Construction. Go see Reverend Joel."

After perfunctory introductions, Reverend Joel walks me over to a ditch and describes my task. I'm ditchdigger for the maintenance department.

"Dig down past these electrical wires to find where the water pipe makes an 'L' turn. When you find that, ask me for further instructions."

Thank Buddha I'm assigned a loner job. *I need time to think.* Since only minimal talking is allowed during work periods anyway, it doesn't much matter. Work is supposed to be done as a form of meditation.

Reverend Joel gives not one second to demonstration, but hands me the pickaxe and shovel, and smiles with a slight bow and a whispered "get to work." I try the shovel first, and the damn ground is hardened clay.

No wonder he left without demonstration.

I grab the pickaxe, raise it up over my back, and swing with all my might. Clunk! It hits the ground and sends shock waves up my arms and down my back. It's a bit titillating. I swing again and crash into the hardened soil. With each swing, I breathe in a great gulp of air and blow out what seems like endless waves of emotional pain. It is exhilarating and cathartic. Hardened bedrock within me dislodges as my ditch widens.

Finally, I have loosened enough earth to begin shoveling. A rhythm develops as I crouch down, shovel in, lift, and hurl the dirt. I'm Paul Bunyan, swinging and puffing and breathing in the pine scent as I blow out great stores of repressed energy.

I can't stay with the flow of my body for long, as my head resumes its worrying.

Great that I brought those rubber gloves. I had no idea I'd be doing such difficult physical labor.

I get instant calluses anyway.

If I develop too many muscles, will my rings still fit? I've planned well, but still, what will I do if a nail breaks?

But can't complain.

Can't talk.

Alternating between pickaxe and shovel, I make a small dent in the work at hand, but move past a mountain of my fear.

I'm afraid?

I can't quite acknowledge that yet.

Anger is easier.

I wonder if they know I have anger to express. At HOPE House, we'd give a job assignment based on clinical needs of the patient. Did I need the digging, pounding, and smashing of rock?

Obviously.

I'm trying to do not just a good job, but an impressive job. *I'm sure Reverend Joel will shower me with glowing accolades later.* The ground is hard, a light-sand color, but it gives way to my pounding. I notice a dank, but pleasant, smell arise from the loosened earth as I gain access deep into its bowels. I am entering new territory, and no one has been here since the pipe was initially laid. At one point I notice a small ant scurrying up my arm. Instead of smashing, I lay him gently on the ground. Treated by these monks with such gentleness and kindness, I want to give back the same.

This place is growing on me.

The work period passes more quickly than expected and the physical exertion takes the morning's chill out of my bones. We've been up since five; first meditating, then working by seven, breakfast, meditation, and back to work. *No rest for the unenlightened.*

Just when my digging settles in to a rhythmic pattern, Reverend Joel stops by my ditch to announce, "Time for class."

Not a word about the job I'm doing. I'm sure he'll comment later.

With a quick clothing change and cleanup, I'm ready to race around the abbey to the classroom to relax into learning what this is all about.

My brain will get its much-needed exercise.

My time to shine.

Energized and thankful I didn't leave too soon, I have a little trouble finding the classroom. Finally, I arrive and plop in just a little late to see all my fellow trainees listening attentively to yet another male monk in brown robes.

Some of them are even sitting lotus at this session.

This monk is short, with the same bald head and the same brown robes, but he seems a little nervous, not as centered as the others.

Clearing his throat, he begins. "Today's session will be about moderation. The Buddha had scorned extremes of eroticism or asceticism and recommended that we find the middle path to enlightenment by living an ordinary life."

I'm excited. I've been debating with treatment professionals over rigid versus *laissez-faire* food plans, and I'm writing a book about moderation in recovery.

Great. I'm gonna get my money's worth.

I truly value intellectual pursuits and discussions almost as much as I devalue meditation, which the monks hold in high esteem. For me, the class is over too quickly, and we're sent back to meditate before lunch. I suffer through yet another meditation session. There've only been three since I first arrived.

And I have six times a day coming.

During meditation I cry while my nose twitches and pain pounds in my head. In each session, my mind races around a NASCAR track. But the minute I leave the meditation hall, all thoughts cease. I feel breezy, relaxed, and lightheaded.

So, I'm not getting it the way I think I should, but I am lightening up some. It takes time.

Time for lunch.

I follow others, grabbing a bowl, silverware, and cup, and then scramble with the rest to find a seat, each of us pretending it doesn't matter where we sit. Massive screeching follows as those steel chairs scrape the floor again.

Is this loud irritation our signal to eat?

It is certainly a contrast to the melodious gong that announces meditation. I'm sure there is more psychological interpretation to devise, but I'm too hungry.

I like the seat facing the picture window that offers a crystal-clear view of the mountain.

Everyone but me knows the meal procedures. I follow along. We ritualistically unfold napkins and give *gassho* as each family-style bowl is passed. We give *gassho* before receiving the bowl, then spoon out our serving and bow again as we pass it on to the left. After all are served, a gong sounds and we take silent bites, giving *gassho* before each forkful.

Why, this could be heaven for my anorexic patients who love to perform elaborate rituals over the food they never get around to eating. Eventually, some of these tools will become a cornerstone to my maintaining permanent weight loss.

Wastefulness is considered morally unethical, and all food that is taken must be eaten. There's nowhere private to stow leftovers for later. The other trainees know not to take what they won't eat.

I make a big abbey mistake after breakfast right in front of the kitchen chief. As we stand silently in line to wash our individual plates, I beam proudly and say, "Where can I store the uneaten half of my orange?" I'm feeling terrifically virtuous at not finishing a meal.

Notice the big deal I can make over half an orange. I wasn't saving a pork roast or anything.

As he swoops up my uneaten citrus, the monk scowls and growls about me to someone in the kitchen.

I'm ready to lose it again. Lower lip starts quivering. I am aware how vulnerable and open I am to any feedback.

Here we go. Here come the tears.

My head brews up a fight. A margin of safety has returned as I sense anger and irritation from this man.

I can deal with that.

My head starts racing defensively to tell him off.

I didn't know the rules. It's your fault.

Instead, I just stand quietly and watch. Frozen in front of his dishwashing window, I psychologically leave the scene, remembering all the many meaningless battles I've fought over the years.

According to the Buddhists, the process of awakening involves seeing in stark relief all the areas of your life that haven't been working. In that awareness, you might feel despair, disgust, and sadness.

Well, it's all happening for me right now.

In this loving environment, I'm beginning to see all the paradoxes in my life and all those areas that don't quite measure up. I'd been so concerned about achieving and proving myself in the world and accomplishing great pioneering things in a very few years. *For what?*

No one cares here. In this cloistered environment, it's more important that I pay attention to not wasting food or not taking more than my share and being aware that the planet needs all of us to remain conscious. In fact, it's continuous awareness, paying attention, and staying present and alive that are the gift and burden of being human. And I have wasted so much time in pursuit of being the top-of-the-heap superhero. All of my efforts were expended in the service of a fearful ego so that I could avoid feeling like a total failure and an inadequate, scared little rabbit.

Is either of those necessary? The truth lies somewhere in between.

I will find my way into mediocrity, daring to be average.

All those years of therapy and training had helped me see the root causes of my competitive striving. My own fat and furious disposition germinated in a home where both parents repressed their own constant fear, pain, and sadness. Their generation didn't talk about deep feelings. They only knew how to express anger. I carried their sadness for them. And no matter how cute and precocious I was, I couldn't fix them. I compensated for this perceived inadequacy by developing a winning personality to use as I went out into the world to win friends and influence people. But then I'd come home to hear, "You've got them all fooled. They can't possibly know how rotten you really are."

Believing from an early age that I was really "no damned good," I walked out into the world seeing and creating my own violence and violation. It's so difficult to avoid hurting self or others. Sadness and pain are just unavoidable.

But who's to blame?

In medicine, the Hippocratic oath admonishes us to "never do harm." The prescription in this monastery is to try to do no harm to any living thing. Facing the difficulty of that prospect, I'm anxious to make small talk with fellow trainees.

I'm anxious to start commenting on these ideas and this experience.

I want someone to see that I tried hard to be good, but screwed up anyway. I want to rant to someone that "the kitchen monk hurt me."

Doesn't he know that I just want to be a good kid? I want to know all the times to bow and to whom. I want to dig the deepest ditch, swoop with the lowest bow, and eat the fullest orange. But I just can't. Instead, silence is the golden rule. I don't say a word.

Silence.

Clearly, I cannot tolerate anything less than perfection. Attached to my need for a perfect image, I will be given innumerable chances to flunk out.

By bedtime, I am resigned to wandering through this place without being appreciated or receiving any praise. I will just *be*.

In a brief twenty-four hours, I have managed to survive and sit in stillness through all the meditation sessions, albeit from my high perch on the bench. I have become acutely aware of sensory input—from quiet gongs of meditation bells to screeching chairs on dining room floors, to the rich smell of earth inviting me to enter deeper. I've watched calluses sprout on my fingers and felt "moderation" ideas sprout in my cerebellum. I have absorbed the security offered by these monks and their structure, and though shocked by the kitchen monk's judgment, I have not diminished my resolve.

Exhausted by nightfall, I tumble into bed with no more energy to cry.

On day two, dressing becomes easier and I can do it faster. I stand upright to put on my prayer skirt while the others are squirming to get dressed while still inside their sleeping bags. "We try not to offend ourselves or others," Reverend Muldoon's words echo.

Well, the hell with that. I've lived a lifelong struggle with obesity, full of shame about my body, stretching hand towels in high school gym classes across rolls of pubescent fat.

So now I should cover up and worry about someone viewing my sleek, slim torso? Offensive? Disturbing someone's practice? Give me a break.

My concession to this monastic modesty is to dress quickly, albeit standing.

Right after morning prayers we are sent out into the freezing cold to line up for work details. The crisp, cold essence of pine needles seeps up my nose as the morning work assignments are called.

"Maureen Richter, who is new today, will work with Judi Hollis for the maintenance department."

Why had they announced my last name? I'm here for an anonymous private retreat. Why are they even giving me a helper? I was doing quite well by myself.

I'm back in the ring.

Maureen wears all the right gear: hiking shoes, baggy pants, a thick pink sweater, and green fleece hat. She is short, with pixie-cut, curly brown hair and a smile that says, "I'm at peace."

I catch her eye and whisper, "I'll show you to the toolshed to get further direction from Reverend Joel."

I pray she's on a different assignment. My head screams, "I want to be alone." I'm sure there's room for only one pick and shovel at *my* ditch.

Guess what? She's assigned to help me.

Damn.

We walk silently and then she asks, "Didn't you give a training presentation at a hospital in San Bernardino last week? I recognized your name."

Clenching teeth, staring straight ahead down the path, I can't decide how to respond.

Caught. I've traveled 600 miles to the top of a mountain to get away from my life. I'm finally settling in to being a newcomer, accepting that I have nothing to do or say but learn. And then, this.

I start laughing. "I don't believe it." I laugh harder and louder. "I just don't believe it." Maureen catches on immediately and laughs with me.

She leans over conspiratorially. "I hope it doesn't make you uncomfortable. I can understand how you'd want to be away from your roles and responsibilities. I just wanted you to know

I thought it was a great seminar and I can really see how your treatment ideas reflect much of what is taught here at the monastery. This is my sixth summer here. My husband and I have been meditating for many years and we incorporate Buddhism into our work as therapists."

I have such a warm, ironic giggle bubbling up and just waiting to escape from my pursed lips.

This is the best cosmic joke ever.

I draw furtively closer to her and whisper, "I try to get away from my professional roles so I can be in a position of learning rather than teaching."

Then I immediately start teaching.

I tell of my struggles: how my center is like this monastery, but how difficult it is to justify within a medical model. I go on sharing my debates about mechanistic, standardized recovery programs teaching "adjustment" versus my more spiritually oriented program of "expansion."

I'd love to rattle on and on.

This is my first conversation, and on my turf, yet.

Something stops me. I explain to Maureen that it's probably best to avoid such discussions. "I'm happy you like my work. I feel guilty talking during work period."

"Me too," she smiles, shrugging her shoulders and giggling like, "We're so, so bad."

However, I keep talking. "I've been quite shaky since I got here. I cry all the time. I see there's a lot for me to learn if I can just stick it out."

"I cried during my first week, too," she counters. "Each time we return here, I find myself getting anxious and queasy during the drive up. There's something inviting and repelling about the experience. I do like the quiet time and the loving people."

We agree not to mention things back down in the world again.

As it turns out, Joel assigns us to the same ditch. Our further "minimal" conversation involves positions for digging, who'll wield the axe, who'll heave on the shovel, and how it seems we'll have to dig much deeper. Very soon it is time for meditation again.

I see that the schedule is difficult because we need so many costume changes.

I could really help them with this. I can understand that they want us to alternate meditation with work and then study, reading, eating, rest, and work. This constant shifting of focus keeps us a bit off balance and open. This makes us resort to using different energies and abilities.

I am very comfortable with my brilliant, albeit silent, comments.

But there are flaws in the schedule. Don't they see how difficult it is to run halfway around the abbey, take a sink bath, change into a skirt and slipper shoes, race back to the classroom, bowing en route, remove shoes, bow, and arrive fresh and on time?

Trainees and monks turn the cloisters into the Indianapolis Speedway and make scheduled events loosely on time. Of course, everywhere, at every shrine, I have to bow. I also learned that as I went through the day, whenever the spirit moved me, it was a good idea to bow. I wanted to do my very best to follow the bowing rules.

Let's not forget that no one asked for my opinion on scheduling. They're certainly missing out on a lot of valuable expertise here. I've been organizing therapeutic communities since 1967. Boy, I sound like all the nursing director patients who came through HOPE House and wanted to devise new charting procedures to make things more "efficient." It is so difficult to move from the helper role to that of the person being helped.

The mind likes its comforts.

Mine quickly races to its lowest common denominator during meditation sessions: "What am I going to wear?"

Quickly surmising that three-quarters of what I've brought is unacceptable—loud, sexy, or inadequate—I have to juggle what I have left for classes, meditation, meals, and work assignments. There are also the rest and reading periods to consider, as well as the hourly weather changes that go from sweltering heat to foggy, cold, and damp. Even more complex than what to wear is how to transport the changes from the luggage room around the cloister to the bathhouse cubicle in as few return steps as possible. Timing is everything. Each outfit has varying requirements and necessitates alternative advanced planning.

If only I had my own room with a closet, I could really settle down to meditating.

On the third day the temperature drops below freezing, forcing me to bring out my suede, fur-lined hunting jacket. Why hadn't I considered that these vegetarian, "do no harm to any living thing" monks might find this jacket ghastly and offensive? I'd never given that a thought as I'd packed, instead musing that the jacket had a rugged and mountaineering feel to it.

It's always about image. Would it help if I told them I bought the jacket used at the Rose Bowl swap meet, that I was not the first owner or initial purchaser, and that I would never custom-order such carnage? Wrapped sheepishly in dead hide, I wend my way around the cloisters. No one says a word to me, but I cringe whenever I catch anyone glancing at my furry lapels.

Don't some of them wear leather shoes? Isn't that a real fur hat covering that shaved dome?

I grasp for straws.

Who cares? It's not about me. No one has time to sit in judgment of me. All monks seem to have a busy schedule, getting quickly from one place to the next, their robes swishing along the path, hopefully not brushing any bugs to imminent doom. All are busy racing around the cloister, chasing their own enlightenment.

Part of the morning's class session deteriorates, as so many do, into a heady debate about male-female issues. The conflict is introduced by an elderly woman, dowdy, with scraggly hair, and awful beige "wedgie" shoes.

With raised brow, she peers down the tip of her nose through wire-rimmed spectacles and starts speaking through pinched lips. "I take offense at the scripture's description of 'woman as temptress.'"

Even on this mountaintop, do we have to find yet another campaigner for the women's cause?

I'm livid.

If I didn't feel so new, little, and scared, I'd rejoinder with "Shaved heads, all monks look alike, each is sworn to celibacy, and we're all sleeping on the same temple floor. Do we care at all about sex? Who the hell cares about temptation at a time like this?"

Well, I guess the dowdy old windbag does. I prefer to let these issues lie. I find myself letting the discussion go by rather than attaching myself to any position.

Am I above such attachment? I think it's more that with all my shoveling of real dirt in the ditch, I'm just too tired to transport any more.

After lunch, I have a new job and a new partner. My coworker is Larry, Maureen's husband, who is tall, with reddish hair, and possessed of her same contented, sweet smile that seems to project a "let's wait and see" attitude. I'm more the "jump in and do" type. Our job is demolition. Now we're into something that can well utilize my talents as well as my defects. Let's destroy whatever it is.

Our task is to tear down an old chicken house. I want to make a sarcastic joke to supervisor Joel. "You mean I'll never get to see my ditch again? Ha ha."

Better not say a word, since there's no telling what new plans he could have for me. After all, I still have the nail job to protect.

To do the job right, someone needs to get up on top and start hauling debris and rot from the roof. I watch Larry's hesitation at mounting some of the more precarious beams, so I scurry up them all the faster.

I'm sure my demolition technique is better than his. After all, I've dated enough construction workers to know the two-by-fours will hold me.

I climb to the roof and begin pulling out rotten boards and ripping up tar paper. I marvel at how rapidly and expertly I mount, rip, and toss the boards.

Friendly monks pass, commenting, "It's about time we got rid of that old chicken coop," or "Careful you don't fall through." I keep going.

They are all so timid and cautious. I'm a type T (thrill-seeking) personality.

I wonder if anyone as adventurous as me has been to a place like this. Do any risk-taking souls get to this sort of place, or is it just fearful, timid creatures who want to retreat from the world and its struggles? Could any of them be as successful as I am out in the real world? Do these monks have any idea who they're dealing with?

Promptly, while my mind races with self-congratulation, I jump up to the top of a rickety beam, lose my footing, and, despite grabbing at clumps of air and a stray piece of tar paper, *whoosh,* I fall through the roof.

Bam! My fall is stopped as I find my crotch straddling a two-by-four. No harm done. I landed squarely on my base plate.

Ouch. Damn, that hurt.

Still concerned with looking good and not showing fear or pain, I laugh it off and resume working.

Larry continues his slow plodding. I settle in to doing the same. My perineum is sending out vibrations to the periphery, gently begging, "No more fun and games."

Later in meditation sessions, I start settling in with self-satisfaction. *Wardrobe is in order. All planned out.* Even though I have no room to call my own, I become territorial about *my* meditation bench and *my* seat with a view in *my* dining hall. My little sense of the jokester is coming back, and I start to see the humor of my situation.

I might even get to like this place.

At dinner, my appreciation for food has returned—fueled, I'm sure, by the colder weather blowing in. Self-satisfied, secure, and gaining a sense of more control, I enter the dining hall contemplating plopping into my mountain-view seat to chow down.

Instead, I find that a new monk has changed my seat.

So much for my mountain view.

When you get too attached, it's got to go.

With that, I become fully committed to staying the whole week. I see that I'll be able to endure whatever comes my way. I see that what I want is not all that important. I don't even mind bowing to the other trainees in our overcrowded, silent bathhouse. I can't help wishing, though, that instead of my bright maroon Betty Boop beach towel, I had brought something beige or light blue. Then I could fit in instead of calling attention to myself, causing distraction at every turn. It seems that no matter how I hang Betty out to dry, her cleavage calls out to every stall.

Why had I never seen this aspect of myself before—this defiant, attention-seeking, tough, and "oh-so-different" self? Where have I been? The good news is that the attention-seeking part of me has produced a gifted public speaker and entrepreneurial innovator. The bad news is that such a needy person is sometimes a major pain in the ass.

FOUR
Keeping the Competitive Edge

Day four.

It's been three days without a shower, doing heavy labor, and I still don't even stink. Well, at least *I* don't think so. Each day I debate taking free time for a shower or a walk in the woods to be alone. Amazing how priorities change. At home, I'd surely shower. Here I crave the lonely woods.

I need rest.

I'm not getting much sleep at the abbey. The temple floor is not conducive to a restful respite. The extremely high ceilings and sparse furnishings create a great cavern of echoing howls. One night, I'm awakened by loud snoring from across the temple floor. At midnight, following the worst bout of bellowing snores, a creeping suspicion arises that the offender could be me. Even though I'm sure I'm not the snorer, in the morning, just in case, I bow even lower to my fellow trainees.

Eventually, I find the snorer turns out to be Mrs. Wedgie-wearing feminist, Margaret, whom I've now diagnosed as "seemingly borderline."

I think Margaret attends these retreats in lieu of seeking professional psychiatric help. I find her especially irritating in class sessions. She constantly asks "me, me, me" questions about "my, my, my" "feelings, feelings, feelings."

This is not psychotherapy! I'd learned in my previous progressions down this spiritual path that we are most judgmental of the defect we've just given up.

Hmmm, so Margaret reminds me of me?

Maybe I should discuss her condition with one of the monks. I could outline some inherent dangers of her hiding out here. Maybe they could counsel her to seek professional help.

I smile at myself. There's really no way to predict that psychotherapy would work for her any more than what she is already doing.

I decide to stop judging her, and instead enter the mouth of the dragon. I will practice changing *my* behavior and *my* attitude. I'd been preaching this wisdom to others: "The only person you can really affect and change is yourself. The only way to improve past negative behavior is to take a corrective opposite action."

I decide to keep quiet, moving toward what offends me.

At bedtime on my fourth day, I pull my sleeping mat right up beside Margaret. What a new opportunity for growth.

Don't complain, don't explain. Just do it.

When the snoring starts, instead of nudging her to turn over, I simply move my pillow to divert the airway between us. I'm ready and willing to endure her constant roar. I've accepted the fact that it will last through the night and, like the song says, "I will survive." Instead, she turns over on her own, to coo like a baby.

Waking up to day five, I find myself bowing to the mountain and the courtyard fountain each time I pass. It's not required, but I am so appreciative when facing them. *Uh-oh, it's happening . . . that gratitude thing.*

When Larry and I pull down the last wall of the chicken house, I finally get that longed-for, approving smile from Reverend Joel. "I'm surprised and amazed at how quickly you've finished."

Joel's not wearing robes, but has on jeans and a tight white T-shirt that hugs his muscles. He stands, leaning back with a right hip thrust forward. Taking in his sexy stance, I'm catapulted back to my preteen Pachuco phase, when I walked the train tracks to Russell City with my friend Arlene. Juan Torres and his grease-slicked pompadour buddies offered flirtatious catcalls from his maroon, low-rider '49 Mercury.

Just the memory brings a slight flip.

I think I've been here too long.

Joel offers us a reward for all our hard work. "You can now separate reusable boards and planks from firewood. Take one stack to the kitchen boiler and the other to the boneyard."

This "boneyard" houses a vast assortment of cinder blocks, bathtubs, chicken wire, rubber tubing, and aluminum siding. Monks before us have been collecting every piece of material that might ever be used again in countless incarnations to come.

Reverend Joel always seems to be laughing at us. He is more casual than the other monks. He rarely bows *gassho* upon greeting and departing, and he seems to make jokes often. Actually, all the monks seem to be having fun most of the time. There's always a slight giggle when they talk. It may be that I like him because of my previous history with construction types. Joel seems more the irreverent steelworker who could whistle or catcall to pretty girls from high up on a girder.

Nail breakage becomes more of a reality as my enthusiasm for this work increases. There's one ready to pop, but I've been "borrowing" Band-Aids from the dispensary. I need more. I take them with permission, of course, but I lie about my need. I intimate that I have a cut when it's really to bolster the nail from an anticipated cut I'll have later.

I'm still getting away with little pockets of dishonesty.

I even lie when trainee Ken loans me dishwashing gloves he's brought to the abbey because he's allergic to detergent. "Oh, me too. I'm also allergic." I just can't let them know who I really am. I wonder if they've figured it out anyway. I wonder if they've even bothered to care.

At lunch, senior trainees, those who've attended many retreats and are more committed, act as food servers. I guess it's important to have gentler, more positive and evolved souls near the kitchen. Energy carries, and if it is too negative, it could upset many stomachs.

I'm out on construction where I can do very little harm.

On this last day before departure, I have requested an individual counseling session. These *sanzen* sessions are for discussing personal issues that emerge during the retreat. They are voluntary and must be requested.

My interest in personal counseling is awakened in the morning's class in which we discuss the Buddha's struggles with schisms among his followers. "Buddha gave his wisdom with an open hand, cautioning all to take it or leave it. He told his followers, 'Don't believe what I say unless it matches your own experience.'"

His teachings appealed to doubting Thomases and skeptics like me.

Thinking about my treatment message and the rifts among my "followers," I wanted to know if separation pain is an inherent and unavoidable part of the human condition. I request a *sanzen*.

Reverend Angela, my assigned counselor, greets me on the path. She is about five feet seven with a sylphlike frame in a thin brown smock, draped so she looks like a Roman goddess. Her jet-black hair is partially grown out for a home visit, and she looks like Gina Lollobrigida in that Burt Lancaster and Tony Curtis movie *Trapeze* from the 1950s.

I suspect names for *sanzen* are drawn anonymously by lot, but as I present my concerns, she seems to *know* me. I begin with that separation/individuation issue, trying to impress her a bit with my expertise as a family therapist and addiction specialist. As I humble myself to ask for advice, I want to make sure she knows with whom she's dealing.

"I am interested in learning more about how to deal with separation and loss. Just like mothers have to watch their kids defiantly struggle to leave the nest, would we see the same individuation process in all of life? Does it have to hurt?

"Buddhists seem to have one answer to all life problems: meditate. What about all the feelings? Didn't the Buddha ever hurt? Didn't he feel doubt when criticized? Didn't he feel sad? Didn't he want to give up?"

I spare her most of the details of my personal history, but keep going for an answer to how to feel less pain. "How can Buddhism relieve my suffering?"

She lets me finish and then breathes in fully, allowing herself what seems like an eternity before answering. "Meditation helps one get an acquaintance with center. We have to feel at peace at our own center, so that we are not pushed and pulled by outside stimuli like gossip and negative criticism. It doesn't mean that you won't feel.

"In fact, more enlightened beings often feel more than others do. They see the broader perspective of what is happening. They are often more invested, being fully alive and participating in life. They will notice, see, and feel *more*.

"Buddha resisted becoming a teacher, seeing that there was so much misunderstanding in life. He saw that stating one's views was a setup for attack. Knowing this, he still had to honor his incarnation. He spoke his truth."

"Wow! Just what I need to hear."

I'm a Buddha in my own mind.

With Angela's words, I feel renewed courage to reenter the psychobabble fray. No matter how gently I try to present my new ideas about eating disorders as a disease, for which addictive treatment is effective, no matter how much I preach that moderation is needed with food, as well as in the rest of life, I invariably receive both accolades *and* biting criticism. I am neither armored nor prepared to realize "it goes with the territory."

Throughout my public career I'd found that most people hear exactly what they want to hear. What I had to say was not all that important. Everyone has their own personal agendas anyway—

especially when it comes to the great American diet debate. After one of my speeches, I found two equally vociferous critics arguing with me that:

1. "You don't have anything else to say besides supporting twelve-step programs; and

2. "You don't support the twelve-step programs enough."

I had to learn to diminish my own self-importance. My job was only to deliver the message. Audience members would each do whatever they wanted to do with it. Just like my first appearance on that high-profile afternoon talk show.

It had happened a few years earlier. As word of my new center spread, I was invited to do television appearances outside Los Angeles. I traveled to New York, Connecticut, and then Minneapolis, where I was invited to debate the author of a book titled *Responsible Bulimia*. The producer of a local Minneapolis morning show had liked my no-nonsense style when he'd booked me on *The Sally Jesse Raphael Show* the year before.

He called in a panic. "I really need your help. We need someone strong enough to really take this guy on. He's lost a lot of weight vomiting, and he's encouraging young women to do the same as a healthy and effective strategy. I can't offer you any compensation, but we'll fly you first class, pick you up in a white stretch limo with bar, and put you up in a suite at the Four Seasons."

Even without the perks, I gladly took on the challenge. What a terrible message. I had to speak out against it.

I did well on the show, speaking gently but firmly, hoping to get this man to see that his vomiting would eventually do him in. He ignored me then, but years later he finally entered treatment to address his eating disorder.

The assistant producer of that Minneapolis show had moved to Chicago to help launch a new female-hosted talk show to compete with Phil Donahue. She called, asking me if I would be willing to appear on it. "We want a popular topic as we are launching this show into the national limelight. We'll title the show 'Diet Failures.' We will have the host and everyone in the audience discussing all the things they've tried that haven't worked. Then, for the last segment, you'll come on as the expert and tell them what really works and why."

Hosanna!

I was stoked. My fantasy life mushroomed: *Now that's the way to use my talents. Everyone will be complaining and whining, and then I'll arrive in the last segment to present* the answer. *All arms will rise heavenward as bodies dive to the floor. They'll sing in unison: "Thank you . . . thank you. You've saved us from obesity, from our lives of gluttony and sloth, to awaken again into the eternal light of the slim. By Jove, we think she's got it."*

That's the show in my head.

Here's how it really goes:

With gorgeous makeup, outfitted to look slim and colorful, I wait in the green room watching the first segments reveal all the drama of failed attempts at weight loss. The whole time I fidget in anticipation, preparing for what will be my glorious entry.

Let me at 'em, coach.

At last—my entrance.

The host asks, "So tell us, Judi. What's the answer?"

"Well, you see, it's a disease, and . . ."

"Oh stop. No way is it a disease."

(Remember, this was 1982 and no one was really taking the eating problem as seriously as I was back then. I was so naive.)

The host stands at the sidelines, motioning, revving up the audience to disagree with me. People yell, and she waves them on.

I try to get in a few words here and there, answering the jeering crowd quietly with a smile. I feel myself tighten into a ball as it seems like my sphincter has floated up to my throat.

I keep smiling.

The host eggs them on. "Audience, don't you think it's a cop-out to call it a disease?"

I am smiling, but livid. I want to find the producer, wring her head off, and scream down her throat, "Why the hell did you invite me onto this show? You know what I'm about. You know my message. Why this?"

Instead I smile some more.

Finally the ordeal is over. I shake hands with the host and her staff and keep smiling. "Thanks so much for this great opportunity."

I keep on smiling as I squeeze in my butt for fear I'll mess my pantyhose.

I fly back to L.A., vowing never to do TV again.

The next day the producer with the talk show calls. "We'd like to have you back."

"No, thanks. I think it's a bad idea."

"No, listen. We got calls saying, 'Why didn't you let her speak?' We want you on to better explain your position. We'll cook up something for after the first of the year and you can do the show however you like. We'll let you produce it, and bring on some patients and present any angle you want. You can focus on that mother-daughter thing. The public really wants to hear from you and we'll let you speak."

Well, that doesn't sound like a bad idea at all. Everything my way? I'll be totally in charge, controlling, having all the power? Producer, yet? What's not to like?

The next two shows go much better, and my television career is launched.

Enough reminiscing and living in the past. Time to get back to work at the abbey.

After my *sanzen* session, as I return to sorting wood stacks, I can't help thinking: *I feel sorry for the poor bastard who'll have to pull out all the nails in these "reusable" boards. I know Larry and I will sort and stack well, and leave the messy drudgery of nail pulling to the next load of victim trainees.*

Just when I'm gloating about how sublime it is to be getting away with something, Reverend Joel stops to admire our stacks. "You two have worked so fast, and I'm impressed. You can now pull all the nails, screws, bolts, and hinges out of the reusable boards."

So our reward is more work, and screwed work at that?

Why are we trying to save all this junk? Oh, I know: because we're not wasteful.

I immediately decide I've miscalculated on some boards. They're not all really "reusable." I want to re-sort my piles and throw the difficult ones into the "firewood" pile.

I'm pissed again. *You don't get away with anything around here.*

Buddhists will tell you that your karma will come. I'd been saving these boards for the next shift. Instead they end up piled right in front of me.

I sure wish lunchtime would come. Gotta get away with something. Food's the way to win.

When lunch finally rolls around, I eat ravenously and quickly, finding it hard to bow between each bite.

Late in the afternoon, Reverend Joel brings us a miracle nail-puller tool. *Doesn't he realize we'd been struggling all morning?* I've already overeaten with resentment, only to now get rescued after the fact. So much of my food obsession is about impatience and an inability to wait.

Now, armed with proper equipment, Larry and I move along speedily. *Boy, how many times have I asked a man to fix something and been told, "I didn't bring the right tools"?* I always felt sure this was some carpenter's cop-out. Now I see how important it is to have the proper implement. Given time, I'm sure to extrapolate some great new psychotherapeutic law from this. Something about building the right toolkit or being up a creek without a paddle or . . .

Instead I joke, "Reverend Joel, where were you when we needed you?" I feel as if I'm a construction master as I use the new tool to rip off a cumbersome hinge with ease. He answers softly, and not at all apologetically, "I thought of it, but then got distracted. Sometimes it takes a bit of time to execute what I think up."

"Too much meditating, I guess," I chuckle, self-satisfied with my cute little barb. "Ha, ha," I continue under my breath as both Larry and Joel remain silent.

Oops!

They stare at the ground. Perhaps they're embarrassed for me and my inappropriateness. I wanted to play.

Next shift I'm reassigned to work alone washing the outside of the temple. Larry will have to stack iron pipes without me.

I wonder if he'll work as efficiently without my competitive edge to spur him on.

I take on temple washing with the same zeal I had for my other tasks. I have brilliant ideas on how the task can be enhanced and more efficiently completed. I keep these ideas to myself, realizing, as if in a lightning zap from heaven above, "There will always be more work." I have passed through competition, showing off "helpful suggestions," looking for accolades and ego gratification, to settle down to doing the work just because it needs to be done.

The Buddhist teacher Shunryu Suzuki Roshi instructed, "When you wash the rice, wash the rice."

Later, I'm assigned to dusting shelves in a storeroom. I encounter two gigantic daddy longlegs spiders that have built elaborate webs. I'm sure there's some Buddhist mandate against squishing these creatures. After consulting the monk in charge, I learn how to address such matters.

Catch the little buggers in a cup and carry them out to the garden to a new abode in the ferns. Bow to all concerned. Then eradicate the webby results of their previous hard work.

I'm beginning to enjoy working more consciously, respecting all living things. I'm gaining more and more respect for myself in the process.

At lunch, I'm reassigned to a window seat.

Once again I fall madly in love with my cloud-covered mountaintop. Each day and each hour the view changes as clouds drift by and sunbeams emerge or retreat. But the mountain is always there, steadfast and secure. I know now that that secure place is what we seek in meditation. You have to get down to solid bedrock. I'm sure it'll be a while before I hit pay dirt.

More changes. There's an extra reading assignment tonight. This will cut into the time I had planned for sitting in the woods. *Why didn't they assign it sooner so I could plan better? How could they expect us to catch up? I know it was some of that "be here now" stuff, but I wanted to* be there then. No one checks on whether or not you do the reading assignment.

I notice that whenever surprised, my first defense is to complain. People here are operating independently of my timetable. When faced with change or surprise, all I can do is squeeze up and congeal and whine. Before reveling in my complaints, I hadn't bothered to see that the assignment was only three pages long. As it turned out, of course, I found time to get the three pages read and also go to the woods. I fight windmills in my mind. It's amazing how quickly these little fits of righteous indignation fizzle out. But sometimes I eat over them instead of waiting. Buddhists say, "Attachment breeds suffering."

And on the seventh day, she rested.

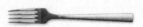

My "old-timer eyes" fill up with tears as I contemplate my last day at the abbey from my present-day vantage point. I'd been waiting to take a picture of the snowcapped mountain, but it clouded over. *Anyway,* I tell myself, *my camera is packed. It's not* beschert, *not meant to be.* Rules are more relaxed for the last day, and we can be more casual around the cloister. Quiet conversations are allowed. Meeting up with Reverend Penelope on the path, I thank her for helping me to the bench that first night of "stilt legs." She responds with "I'm so proud of you that you stuck it out."

How can she say such a thing to me? I feel my eyes begin to tear up again. *I'm a renowned psychologist and lecturer. She's talking like I'm a little five-year-old girl. Maybe I am that five-year-old, and she's known all along.* I've needed the week to catch up.

I am beginning to feel grateful. Before coming to the abbey, I was well practiced in getting my way, knowing what I wanted and how to get it. I definitely knew what I would not tolerate. By not getting my way, I learned that I really can endure. I'm glad I was ready to stick it out, because now I find myself bowing at mountains and fountains.

I have just spent a long week seeing in graphic high relief my attachments to life as I know it. My obsession with orderly accumulation of clothes and mixing and matching of outfits is something I've been suffering from for years. Since I've lost weight and found that so many clothes look good on me, I've amassed an extensive wardrobe, rationalizing that my career requires dressing well, and sale bargains make it worth the price. In reality, this has become a form of attachment for me to bind my anxiety.

Who am I dressing the doll for at Shasta Abbey?

How can I justify the hours in meditation plotting trips to the luggage room?

I will have to put in quite a bit more meditating on a regular basis to discover what that obsession helps me avoid.

Instead of the room of my own, I found a quiet place within and a place in the wild to claim for myself. I could watch "wedgies'" snoring subside when I accepted it and stopped trying to control. Most of all, I'd found a compassionate love for myself and others struggling with the human condition.

I explained to Penelope, "I think it was great that I was immersed midway into the retreat. There was no chance for my head to fight the system.

"I was coming to the abbey to learn, not to grow. I wanted to stand back and watch, tsk-tsking through pursed lips. Instead, it was such a shock to my system that I just moved into survival mode, slowed down to one day at a time, and let the process unfold."

I hug her and laugh about how adamant I'd been against the bowing. "When I wasn't insisting on having my own room, I was complaining about the bowing."

She looks at me in deadly earnest and says, "When the bowing dies, Buddhism dies."

I feel a fragile fear of returning to my world. I don't want to in any way injure myself or others. I know that is impossible, so I'll try to make the best of it. Before departure, I place a stick of incense at the attachments shrine and say a deep personal prayer, hoping to give up more. As the incense wafts up my nose, I notice that I am wearing my smallest Ralph Lauren jeans, silk blouse, Western boots, and French-manicured nails.

All are intact.

But after all, who's counting?

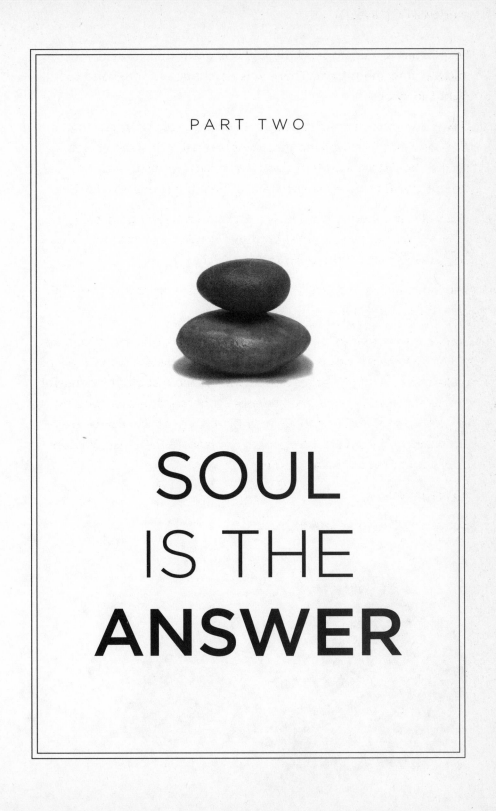

PART TWO

SOUL
IS THE
ANSWER

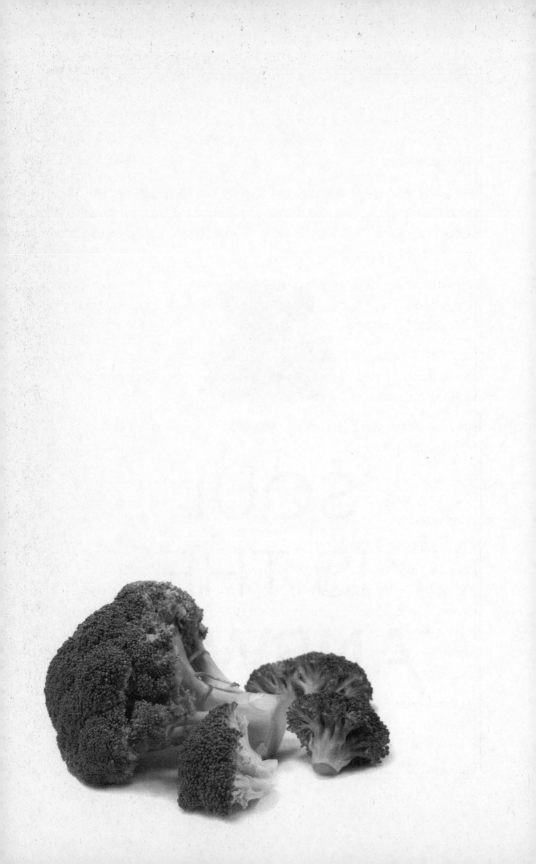

ONE
Prayer Changes the Pray-*er*

I return from the abbey motivated to create more time and space in my life. I move key people into positions of higher responsibility at HOPE House. Becoming more of a motivator/ trainer, I don't fully realize yet that I'm actually freeing myself up to take my act on the road. But within a month, I'm offered recurring segments on a national TV show. That generates other appearances. I earn entrance into the Screen Actors Guild (SAG). I also get more lecture bookings, and for higher fees. Basking in media exposure, full of righteousness, I accept the abundant pump for my ego.

This is an ironic contrast to the way things were thirteen years earlier. In the early 1970s—while still bingeing on food and fighting with my alcoholic husband—I'd been feverishly working to acquire my own TV show. I ran around Hollywood, tap-dancing and impressing others, selling myself, and overeating. But when I faced the time and effort necessary to stop eating compulsively, I gave up all aspirations of appearing on the tube, instead focusing on curbing my food intake. After I entered recovery, I spent my time each morning boiling two eggs and slicing grapefruit.

Now, in the 1980s, with more opportunities coming my way and with little effort on my part, I see that I don't want the daily pressure of my own show. It's easier being a guest. I say my piece about my specific area of expertise and then leave. That's honestly all I have to offer. I don't have enough to say to justify my own forum day in and day out. So, many pounds later, as TV spots come to me, I see that letting go of the TV-show dream and holding it with a "looser hand" brought better and more appropriate results.

Continuing with lecturing, writing, and "tubing," I also begin serious study of the meditative path with Shinzen Young, a Los Angeles monk teaching from the *Vipassana* school of meditation. And he looks like I think a monk should look. He's a short Jewish guy with a gnarly, kind face and seems to be in a daze most of the time. He speaks softly and clearly and with great assurance. I'm inspired with confidence that Shinzen can help me find a way to adopt Buddhist principles into my everyday life. I verify that he truly is a monk. Why, he'd even had an audience during the pope's visit to L.A. It doesn't get much holier than that.

Along with a group of other therapists, I sign up for Shinzen's weekly class. We're all trying to integrate Eastern philosophies into our Western psychology practices. We gather together because many of us have seen that therapy is much more an art than a science, and that rather than curing illness, we are teaching and welcoming sufferers into enlightenment.

Despite professional connections with these other students, I again feel like a fish out of water. They've all obviously spent more time meditating than I have. Many seem well versed in every form of growth group from Brugh's *Joy's Way* to the est holes of Calcutta. During class breaks, I eavesdrop on tales of new body work gurus in town or marathon workshops. All share intimate, personal revelations, busy owning and explaining "internal processes."

Have I mistakenly scheduled myself into a gastroenterologists' conference?

Each week I sit through the breaks, talk to no one, and anxiously await pearls of wisdom from Shinzen. I rarely speak and make few friends. But other than an occasional, slight, hesitant smile to the gracious hostess who welcomes the class to her Westwood home to enjoy her masks, Buddhas, and rugs from her many trips round the world, each night I leave early and don't find any *sangha* there. (*Sangha* means "community" and refers to learning with a congregation of like-minded fellow meditators.)

I do, however, learn to sit on the *zafus* for twenty-minute stretches at a time. That's a tremendous feat, though after each session I hobble home. I feel satisfied that I've surrendered and given up my insistence on having things my way. After a few months, Shinzen asks one evening at the end of class, "Would anyone wish to share what you've been experiencing in meditations?"

I stammer, "I'm sort of having a bad . . . well, not really sort of . . . I'm having a bad time. I find myself becoming bored and irritable with things that used to excite me. I'm not able to rev up or invest energy in things the way I used to. I'm feeling unsettled. I think I'm depressed."

I was reminded of a time early on, after my first two years of eating moderately and mindfully, when I had experienced this same listless inability to invest in my life. In addiction treatment circles, we have found that relapse tends to be most dangerous after two or five years of recovery. It is this listless, lost feeling that leads many back to their compulsions. Doors seem to close without new ones opening up. For impatient people, feeling trapped in hallways is not a good place to be.

This "hallways" feeling had first appeared in 1975 when I'd lost my initial sixty pounds and was clearly adapting to a new "normies'" (i.e., normal) lifestyle. I had forsaken my childhood and all I'd ever known. All the transitions I'd experienced before as an "army brat" had not bothered me in the least. I'd survived all that with my favorite comforter and protector—food. But without bingeing, life hurt.

Back in the present, Shinzen stares right through me for a brief period and then smiles. "Could you cite an example that illustrates what you are saying *to a certain extent*?" He then explains to the group that "I use that phrase 'to a certain extent' because it is quite helpful in drawing people out. It helps them relax, to give up struggling for the perfect way to express themselves."

I respond, "I find myself at my own lectures feeling bored and disinterested. I have an out-of-body experience as if I'm standing behind my own back and disdainfully complaining, 'Why is she talking that same old crap? Doesn't she have anything important to say? This all seems so meaningless and trite.'"

Jeff, who like me sits quietly at breaks without socializing, popped up with "I have those same feelings at your lectures."

The whole group laughs and I smile warmly at him. His humor helps take the edge off things. *I'd like to get to know him,* I thought.

A bit embarrassed, but more relaxed, I continue, "I've canceled some of my lectures because I can't seem to go on. I also feel useless hanging around my treatment center, saying the same old things to the same old people. Obviously some of this is a bit disconcerting."

Shinzen gives another long, slow smile. "Your experience is quite common. You are in a stage of vast transition. It is quite uncomfortable. The Christian mystic, Saint John of the Cross, who was early renounced and later canonized, advises that 'you seek and ye shall find.' In his *Dark Night of the Soul,* he wrote about such discomforts on the spiritual path. One feels all alone, as if forsaken by God and self. One longs for home and peace. Mystics welcome this longing. In Western psychological terms, this same experience is diagnosed as 'major depression.'"

The class breaks out in laughter, and I join in with "Well, thanks a lot."

Shinzen continues to explain this phenomenon in a way I find healing and comforting. "You are moving from having been a very strong and vital brain-fueled force in the universe, *an actor.* Now you are shifting direction to become more of a channel for other energies from other sources. You are becoming available to transmit energies and messages you previously could not access. It will come less *from* you, but more *through* you."

Wow. That's it. I'll become more intuitive, less ruminative. I like that vibration feeling when it all seems so seamless.

"Well, I have even more," I continue. "While meditating, I'm mostly in 'monkey mind' and have no calming sensations. I'm tense. Then, after the sessions, my body feels so alive, like I'm absorbing everything around me. Sometimes I look at the ground and see it undulating, like I'm watching the earth breathe."

Shinzen reassures me, "Don't worry that you don't feel focused during meditation. It is far preferable to notice life change *off the cushion* than to describe brilliant awareness and images while in meditation, but no life change outside the hall."

"Okay, but I'm confused. From all I know of schizophrenia, with delirious ramblings about supersensitivity and loss of boundaries,

I am concerned. I am now mouthing the same unintelligible 'thin skin,' 'feel too much' complaints I've heard from patients for many years."

This smiling monk does not seem at all disturbed.

"There is nothing to fear here. You are not cracking up. Rumi wrote, 'Give up your drop to become part of the ocean.' You are expanding your boundaries, becoming more a part of the human race, part of all things. You are at sea, beginning to have the sorts of sensations that many go through just prior to their first enlightenment experience."

I guess I'm supposed to feel good about this.

I really don't have a clue what this man is talking about, but I listen intently. His response feels like a reassuring "Stay tuned for coming attractions." But I don't know if I want to buy a ticket just yet. I smile back and say nothing.

I want to tell him more, but am afraid of hogging the group time. I want to tell him there have been some startling moments recently, during which I wondered *who* was talking through my mouth or seeing through my eyes. I found these moments elevating rather than depressing. I decided to stop questioning. Instead, I listen to Shinzen's ending.

"That 'depressive neurosis' in Western terms or 'dark night of the soul' in mystical talk is a necessary rest stop on one's transit through the galaxy. It is important to fully exalt and respect the experience rather than pushing too fast to get through it."

I sense a brief rush of excitement over the uncertainty of not knowing what's in store along with a renewed commitment to see it through.

The day after Shinzen's class, a major producer nixes my appearance on his show because "she's too fat to be talking about what she's representing."

I can't believe it. How shallow and superficial. I wonder if he has an eating disorder. Does he know that part of the problem is in trying to achieve unrealistic body standards? Why can't a person with well-rounded physical attributes represent expertise in this area?

I am livid. I want to kill. I want to eat!

In that order.

So that's another door slammed shut. It looks like a clear sign to me. *I'm supposed to give up this media crap*. I accept that the producer might be right. If I want to talk more of this talk, I might have to lose the ten pounds I've regained over the past few years. I still look normal and attractive, a far cry from my all-time high, but not bone-thin, either. If I want to play in that medium, though, I have to accept that everyone photographs heavier, and producers still look at the body.

But my body is turning on me in other ways. My recurring backaches return with a vengeance. My Los Angeles yoga teacher gets me a special consultation with his teacher, Shreehardin, visiting from Madras. Maybe he can help.

When we meet, he is rail-thin, wrapped in a plain white cotton tunic covering pencil-thin cotton pants, and wears his glasses dangling at the end of his nose.

He asks me to raise my right leg.

"Now the left, please. Please bend over. Stand up straight and lean backward as far as you can."

While I contort into his recommended poses, he scrawls on his pad, making stick-figure drawings to explain his prescription for me. "First of all, sitting on *zafu* is not good for you. Your back and hips will never accommodate such postures. Also, you must practice better breathing. In yoga, breath is everything. We want you to make long exhales. Notice the arrows on the drawings that indicate when to breathe in and when to breathe out. On your long exhale, I want you to chant the word *MAAAAAAAAA.* Please chant that for me now."

I stall.

"A problem?"

"Well, not really," I say. "It's just that in the US, many of us have issues with our mothers. It could be an uncomfortable conflict chanting to Ma when trying to heal."

"Oh, in India also," he explained. "Many of our ancient stories are of threatening and ghastly mothers. Even today, no one wants to pay for a daughter's expensive wedding and dowry. We have, even in the smallest villages, ultrasound clinics where we ascertain the sex of a fetus. A girl fetus is destroyed by the mother. Over half a million girl babies are thrown away each year."

I guess I should be grateful my mother let me live.

"But this will not be at all about you or your mother. We want you to forget your actual mother. It is unimportant. We merely want you to chant the sound of MAAA . . . AAAA. We want you to feel the vibration of the sound while thinking of Mother Earth, nurturance, and the sun. You can feel thankful for all you are given to experience each day of your life. It is more about gratitude than motherhood. You will practice proper breathing as you chant your MA."

He watches me do a few practice breaths as instructed, dividing the cadence into a long MAAAAAAAAAA followed by a shorter AAH. But I can't block out thoughts of my own mother. Completely unaware of my struggle, he comments, "Very good, now." His voice is deep and melodic and he speaks with an oh-so-fast, slightly British-sounding accent.

"How often and with what regularity will you take on this practice? It is most important that you make a commitment you can live with. Much better than to promise what you cannot deliver."

I am ready to promise him the farm when he turns my body fully toward him and stares squarely right up under my nose. "Commitment is everything. Commitment is the primary tool for transformation. In a moment of lucidity, we make a commitment to a new behavior we think will change us. Then, later, when it comes time for the behavior, time to do a practice, eat an apple rather than a candy or whatever; the old way will always feel like the right choice because it is more familiar, thus easier. The mind will supply many reasons why the old way actually makes more sense. (Twelve-steppers call this "stinkin' thinkin.")

"At such times, all we have to lean on is our previous *commitment* to the new behavior, made in a moment of lucidity. Also, honesty and integrity are important for building confidence. Making commitments that we don't keep is like lying to ourselves, acting without integrity. Therefore, breaking commitments erodes confidence; we stop believing in ourselves. Therefore, from a psycho-spiritual perspective, it is better to honor a commitment to do your new behavior only once a month and keep that promise, rather than to commit to a daily reform and only do it six times a week."

Shree's advice is so convincing that I forget all I've learned about making commitments, that I can only promise for one day at a time. "Okay, Shree, I will do ten minutes a day, minimum twice a week, but only after my next lecture tour."

"As you wish," he says and smiles, jotting down my promise and drawing our session to a close.

With my posture prescription in hand and well practiced in my "Ma-Ah" chants, I meekly inquire, "May I ask about something else?"

"Of course."

"I have been questioning my professional life for quite some time. Do I have a gift and a message to deliver? I really want to know. Am I supposed to continue the speaking and publishing juggernaut?"

Is Oprah waiting?

"Continue as you have been doing. Do only what is comfortable and easy. Do not promote. Let things come to you."

I leave Shreehardin with a smile and a prescription plan of "easy does it."

I know that if I am to embark on a spiritual path, I need to reestablish more discipline in my life. And remember, my back is killing me! I've gained back just enough weight, I guess. I've been eating rather casually, content with my clothes and size, rarely feeling deprivation. I've been spending compulsively, buying myself any trinkets that strike my fancy. As a discount shopper, I know those little forays don't require Debtors Anonymous yet, but I rarely say no to my little cravings. I know it's time to pull in the reins and put my money where my mouth is.

I'll try a twenty-one-day stint of returning to basics, practicing the things I'd learned during my initial weight loss. I'll develop a daily, disciplined food plan, write it down, and share my commitment and intention with a fellow sufferer. I will tell this person exactly what I eat each day, weighing and measuring portions whenever possible. I'd learned earlier that daily accountability with this other fellow traveler makes me think twice about my choices. If the commitment is made only to myself, then I am sure to break it. I can talk myself into anything. But how will I explain deviation from my commitment to another person? At least, having that accountability outside of self gives me a moment of pause. I have to pay attention and think of how to explain my choices.

I commit to working consciously to stay on a weight-loss food plan right up to my next television taping. That would be only a month away, and the month includes the binger's High Holy Day of the year . . .

Thanksgiving.

In AA, they say that New Year's Eve is "amateur night." Thanksgiving is amateur night for overeaters. Amateurs have no idea how the true overeater can eat.

Well, as I'd said when I first started this journey on November 22, 1974 (five days before you-know-what), "You've got to start in the midst of the storm, or you'll never get started at all."

There's never a good time to start change; however, this time surely seems to be the worst. *While beefing up my meditation, I had been beefing down mass quantities of food. I need to curb the portions. Now I'll face meditation with fewer comforts, closer to the bone.*

I call Shinzen for a bit of reinforcement, as I'm still feeling shaky. "You are losing old defenses, becoming like a wire mesh with ever-widening holes. You are not yet at the stage of transparency when these things will sail through without hurting. Later, you will be more permeable and it won't hurt. For now, you experience pain. You struggle as the old ways hold on while the new have not yet blossomed."

I'm standing in the hallways. May as well decorate.

TWO
Channel

Way back in 1976, I'd already had that "channeling" experience Shinzen mentioned. My early experiment with transposing addiction treatment to address overeating was going so well that within a year of starting, I was scheduled to give a speech to the medical committee of Los Angeles's San Pedro Peninsula Hospital to convince them to establish a fully independent hospital service. I was not a doctor yet, only a consulting marriage and family counselor, so I was quite intimidated. I knew these were medical people who wanted to see double-blind studies and positive results from other experiments. But this idea was so new that there were no results to reference.

I decided to gather data from all programs doing similar treatments and combine those ideas to make my case. I found that the Mayo Clinic was teaching some of the exercise programs we were also doing. Nutritionists in other places were adopting parts of the addiction idea, and a few books were cautioning against excesses of sugar. Family systems theory in counseling also fit right in.

I worked on the speech for weeks. In those days before PowerPoint, I made flip charts with graphs and statistics. I practiced each evening, flipping charts and running slides. I was ready. But when the time came, I froze! A half hour before the luncheon, I looked over my notes and panicked. I couldn't remember any of my brilliant points. The words on my note cards came out as gibberish. I didn't even understand a notation where I told myself to flip the chart for my next graph.

Unnerved, I called a spiritual mentor, who advised me to calm down and go inward. She told me to meditate and then ask to be a channel so the message could pass through me. I practically screeched into the mouthpiece, "That crap is fine for you and your meetings, but THIS IS MEDICINE!"

She answered with a timeworn response used by many wounded healers: "Well, that's what I'd do."

You really can't argue with someone's personal experience. Her advice was like the St. Francis prayer recommended in Step Eleven of some of the twelve-step programs. It was just like Shinzen's story about letting things flow through the wire mesh. I didn't trust any of it, but I was desperate. I found a cubicle and actually bowed down to recite the St. Francis prayer, "Let me be a channel of thy peace." Then I mounted the podium and began.

Well, I was thoroughly disappointed. I didn't express any of the passion and excitement I felt for this innovative project. This was my baby, my life's product, my soul, and I gave a totally boring delivery. It all sounded like mush to me. My New York huckster persona was having an out-of-body experience. She stood back near the curtain, screaming at the speaker, "Kick it in, kick it in!" Instead, I continued with a bland and boring lecture devoid of all pizzazz. Finally, I heard applause, so I sat down.

Completely demoralized, I was afraid to come back to work the next day. As I entered the hospital, I was stopped by nurses and techs enthusiastically asking to work on my new unit. It seemed that the doctors loved what I had to say. If I had shown the passion I felt, they might have been put off or afraid I'd lead them down some dangerous path. Instead, some other energy showed up and knew *exactly* what those doctors needed to hear. It wasn't for me to be entertaining. I was there to get the job done. In my confusion, I finally saw that there was more going on than my little head dreamed up. There was also an interaction between me and the audience that I couldn't control. We both had created the event. It was like good sex, only with a crowd.

That lecture was my first experience with channeling and letting go. Buddha said that all human suffering came from our attachment to wanting things as we want them or trying to keep things as they are. To live mindfully, we must go with the flow. Keeping a solid inner core of personal awareness, we ebb and flow with life's changes. Seng-Ts'an, the third Zen patriarch, said, "The Great Way (i.e., the path to enlightenment) is not difficult for those who have no preferences."

Imagine if you had no preferences. Difficult, because, as with most overeaters, you (and I) want what we want when we want it. I trust my head to know what's best for me. At any heightened-awareness state, food is always the first and easiest choice. If only the world could be in my skin, anticipating my needs before I have to express them. That's what the umbilical cord did. There is nothing as responsive today as there was during those good old days in the womb when I was continually fed without having to tug on the plug. It seems to be the human quest to find a womb with a view.

Overeating once filled that bill, but it eventually cost too much. Living without having things always go my way will mean growing into a spiritual adult. I'll be able to live with *enough*?

I'll be able to trust my body about what *full* feels like? Despite professional accomplishments, my eating compulsion periodically still turns on me. It functions as an accurate barometer of my spiritual condition. Elizabeth Gilbert, author of *Eat, Pray, Love,* says she is a better person when she has less on her plate. How apt. When I am piling on too much in my life and want to scream, "Get off my back," my body delivers the message loud and clear. I break out in back pain. A nurse once told me, "One pound on the body feels like ten pounds on the back."

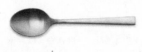

Now that awakened body directs my next level of spiritual growth. "Spinal stenosis," says the orthopedic surgeon. "You've put your body through a lifetime of abuse. Scoliosis developed during your adolescent growth spurt when your enlarged abdomen set you off balance. Your spine grew in crooked, and then carrying all that weight for so many years has caused arthritis in your lumbar and sacral regions. It is called spinal stenosis and basically means that you have excess deposits of bone squeezing in on your spinal cord."

Suffice it to say, "Ouch!"

"We can give you the fentanyl patch that is highly addictive or surgery or physical therapy."

I avoid the patch after hearing from my some of my anesthesiologist patients that it is their most highly addictive drug of choice. I settle for physical therapists who then recommend yoga.

(Funny, I am forced to honor my commitment to Shreehardin whether I want to or not.)

Regular yoga practice becomes a form of meditation for me to unite body and soul. Stretching is better than sitting lotus, which is the worst thing possible for my hips. This way, I can meditate while in the postures and save on time. I start gratefully accepting my body with its stocky contours and its periodic weight gains as both my blessing and my curse.

Even though my yoga practice provides quite enough meditation, I decide to try an introductory, beginner's weekend at the abbey. I might as well try the usual and customary introduction. I'll get my horse before the cart, my ducks in a row, so to speak.

Despite all my best efforts, I still arrive to the abbey late.

At that rickety entrance gate, I am met with smiles and warm welcomes. "Good to see you again."

"How nice you came back."

I'm shocked that they even remember me. I'd been silent throughout my earlier stay. *How do they know me?* Remember, they'd had no chance to observe my winning, witty personality. Reverend Joel is busy fixing the front gate. As we smile, I secretly hope that I'll work construction again and be given another lonely outpost under his not-so-watchful eye.

At dinner, Ken, the blond San Francisco youth who'd loaned me the kitchen gloves during my first summer visit, is now wearing the black robes of a novice monk and his head is shaved. I'd had no idea he was headed for monkdom. He works as a food server. Throughout the weekend I try to catch his eye to smile a little gleam of recognition, but he invariably avoids my gaze.

I wonder about this: *Perhaps as a new monk, he doesn't want contact back with the "other side." Maybe he's on special assignment. Oh, I forgot. Male monks don't look at women directly.*

This guy is serious.

After dinner, Reverend Kincaid approaches. "Judi, you've been here before, so you can skip meditation instruction. You know what to do."

"But I want to savor each new trainee experience. I want to go through it all, just in case there is something I've missed," I plead.

Gluttony?

Kincaid smiles, giving me neither approbation nor further recommendation. These monks operate with an economy of effort. It would all be my karma now.

I willfully sneak into the meditation instruction anyway. All the new trainees are perched on *zafus* listening to a monk explain *zazen* meditation. I quickly amble over to my favorite bench.

I know how many hours will be spent facing those blank walls. Even though I've been sitting on zafus, *I don't want anyone here to know that. Twenty minutes at a stretch with Shinzen's group is fine, but there is no way I'll sit on a* zafu *for two days. Better to "easy does it."*

Is this Zen? All this "grabbing" mentality, wanting all that I want, working to look good and act smart?

Is this what a bodhisattva *would do?*

A *bodhisattva* is someone who has been a practicing Buddhist, become enlightened, gone around the wheel of karma a few times, and had the chance to transcend out and not come back. Instead of escaping the endless wheel of karma, the merry-go-round of birth, suffering, and death, that person decides instead to remain here in the game to help others find the path. *Bodhisattvas* take on their training practices for the benefit of all beings. They keep faith in the abundant universe, staying open and sharing and spreading the word. They believe there will be enough for us all. They vow to work toward the enlightenment of all sentient beings, staying until the job is done. There is not one ounce of selfishness in such a being.

That's not me.

Midway through the instruction, a bearded gent looks up from the floor, his eyes popping out above a large smile of recognition. He mouths a conspiratorial "Hello."

He acts as if we're old friends, but though he looks familiar, I can't place him. "Shh, we're supposed to be silent," I gesture and mouth.

As he looks away sheepishly, I remember him as Leon, a seminar organizer I'd worked with to put on a retreat in Las Vegas. I had told that audience about my stay at the abbey and about "my earliest spiritual experience."

That first spiritual hit had landed on November 28, 1974. It was that last Thursday of the month, the High Holy Day. As a lifelong "grazer," I had never experienced a Thanksgiving Day without bingeing. On that particular morning, I awoke in my fourth day of sugar withdrawals. Crying and shaking, I was sure I just couldn't make it safely through an afternoon buffet at Aunt Myra's house.

And I was bringing a favorite yeast dough.

My husband had just returned from a night out drinking. His atonement involved building bookshelves for my office. After most of his benders, I got a lot of new carpentry work done. We all make our deals.

This time, I was not at all interested in his escapades. I telephoned the new mentor I'd met at my first support group meeting three days before.

She advised me to sit alone and write my feelings. I grabbed a spiral notebook and announced dramatically, imagining back of hand stuck like Velcro to troubled brow, "Howard, do not disturb. I am sequestered to write."

He ignored me.

As soon as I sat down to the desk, a distant memory appeared:

I am five years old, an army dependent living in the wreckage of war-torn Europe. It's Frankfurt, Germany, 1950. Most buildings are still rubble from the war. I am walking home alone from my playmate Claudia's house. We've just been playing "tea party," sitting with cups and saucers and our dolls. Making my way down a tree-lined street with cracked sidewalk, I keep walking, feeling safe and secure, watching the cracks.

I sense a loving voice, reassuring, guiding. She whispers, "Just stay on the path. All your needs are met. There is nothing for you to worry about. You don't have homework. You don't have to prepare dinner. No one needs you. There is no present or future. Just be here now. There are no expectations. All you have to do is walk straight ahead, watching the sidewalk. Look at the trees and smell the air. Keep going straight ahead."

I calmed down and stopped crying.

With that gentle, reassuring memory, my hunger and withdrawals subsided.

After that recollection I vowed to myself, *I think I'll tap into this feeling as often as necessary. For now I'll name this "higher power" Claudia, after my playmate.*

That Thanksgiving I ate dinner like a lady and left Aunt Myra's with dignity, feeling neither longing nor deprivation, but instead gratitude and appreciation. I was no longer fighting food, or myself, by myself. I found a "higher self" to watch over me and help me avoid the "self-destruct" button.

But, now, years later, I seemed to have lost that sense. I'd been lapsing back into self-destruct mode, drifting from my true home. That's why I'd returned to the abbey, where I continue staring down at Leon. He has that look of so many male recent weight losers. His clothes are baggy, still trying to cover up, and he sports a scruffy beard to keep hiding out in plain sight.

But, even though he's at the abbey for himself, I am immediately possessive and resentful. I surmise that I've told too many people about this place and ruined it for myself. It's always about *me*. The abbey would no longer be a safe, anonymous refuge—for me!

Shut up, you selfish brat! I hear that ancient call from the recesses of my mind.

Leon's introduction to *zazen* proves much more dramatic than mine. He eagerly crosses his legs lotus-style, mounts his pillow, and joins others on the floor, staring into his wall. I remain up on my elevated perch, jealous that he, a newcomer, is down there with the lotus limb-locked. Some time into the meditation period, I glimpse him in my peripheral vision, rocking and breathing heavily. I know he must be hurting by now, since my back is getting that slight midspine ache.

Leon's knees must be giving out as he begins to move, snapping his legs apart and crawling over to my bench. Hoisting himself up beside me, he resumes staring at the wall. Instead of assuming the tripod forward lean to gain balanced stability, he plops himself squarely on the back of the bench. His effort completed, and breathing settled into normal flow, he resumes sitting and staring. (Notice where I am focused at this time—I could recite chapter and verse of Leon's experience, as I am totally out of mine.)

Quickly after his breathing normalizes, I hear a resounding thud. Leon falls directly backward off the bench, landing perfectly flat, full head and back on the floor. His legs are still bent at the knee, calves and feet still occupying the space beside me.

Stunned, I break my halfhearted meditation and turn to shake his legs. "Are you okay?"

He's out cold.

Snoring loudly and deeply, his great honks for air echo throughout the cavernous temple.

Are you kidding me?

Reverend Arlene comes over to assist and gently shakes him to consciousness. She whispers to me, "Please help with lowering his feet off the bench to the floor."

I do as told, and then she points me back to my seat to resume *zazen.* Needless to say, I don't easily flow back within, but instead keep all antennae focused on Leon and the muffled conversations between the two monks comforting him. Thankfully, there is a gong to signal the session's end.

The next day Leon stops on the path to tell me about his ordeal. "I'd lost blood from my legs while on the *zafu,*" he chortles. "When I got up, blood left my head and rushed to refill—thus, my immediate passing out." He seems in good spirits and not harmed, and ready to take on the rest of the weekend.

"Oh, I feel so responsible for what happened to you. I wish I'd never mentioned this place."

"Get over yourself, Jude. This is *my* experience."

"Oops. You're right. I guess I would do better to keep focusing on *mine.*"

"By the way," he continues, "how are things working out with your mother? Is she angry about your mother-daughter book?"

How could he bring up my mother in a peaceful setting like this? I never should have shared so openly at his event. I thought what happened in Vegas stayed in Vegas.

I had told Leon's Las Vegas group about a recent intervention trying to get my mother off drugs. Her Aunt Rae had called me, screaming, "Your mother fell in her apartment and broke her arm. Why aren't you back here with her? What are you doing out there in California helping all the *goyim*?"

I quickly set up an intervention at my training group in Los Angeles and flew my mother out, hoping this time she would listen and accept some help. Instead, she went further into drug use, and for years afterward screamed at me, "I'll never forgive you for talking about my drug use in front of all those therapists!" She eventually quit drugs cold turkey when her doctor died from his own overdose.

It was right after *Fat & Furious* was published. There was a lot of promotion, including special segments on *The Sally Jesse Raphael Show*. After watching that particular show, Mom told me with very bland affect, "Oh, it's a good book." A month later, possibly then out of drugs and angry about something unrelated, she turned on a dime and screamed, "You wrote a whole goddamned book about me!"

I screamed back, "The book's not about you. It's about my patients and my work. Does everything always have to be about you?"

In truth, of course the book was about her. It was about us. It was about the struggle between all mothers and daughters. I was compelled to write about that dreaded subject; I showed my best and worst and everyone's pained and doomed ambivalent struggle to connect as well as separate.

No one has ever awakened the same neck-veins-popping, eyes-ablaze, red-faced, fever-pitched, wet-spitted rage that my mother did, nor will any other earthling ever be so intimately focused on *me*. I was one of her many obsessions. She—a battling middle child in a family of screamers, early abandoned by a workaholic mother—had a lot on her plate. She piled mine high as well.

We had some good moments. We laughed a lot as we sat at that chrome-legged Formica table, covered with a greasy oilcloth to catch all the fallen black seeds in dribbled slabs of butter from our oversized kaiser rolls. Gossiping and scheming, we relished talking about other people, picking *them* apart, noting *their* failings, devising plans to make *them* feel bad and make *us* look good.

Such discussions created ravenous appetites. I don't doubt that that tendency to closely scrutinize others' behavior played a part in my choice to become a therapist. I was hypervigilant and aware. Back then, there were few encouraging or complimentary comments that passed our lips. I would have to go to graduate school and later study Buddhism to learn anything about compassion for my fellows or myself.

Sometimes it was great pots of noodles mixed with melted butter and cottage cheese with lots of salt and pepper that fueled our tirades about "those people." Come to think of it, most of our easy times together were greased with butter.

Something crunchy like ten-pound bags of pistachio nuts could keep our psyches occupied and the rage in check. Food helped us stay externally focused, lacking in personal introspection or painful self-examination. Chewing and crunching on popcorn, again with lots and lots of butter, helped us to express the anger. Or the longing we each had, the deep yearning for connection and intimacy, the great unexpressed love and fear, could sometimes be quelled with huge, soothing scoops of ice cream covered with nuts and caramel.

Sex and dirty jokes were always welcome. Mom's favorite was about the woman who calls the record store to see if they stocked a new release, but gets the hardware store instead.

"Do you have *Hot Lips and Seven Kisses*?" she asks.

"No, but I have hot nuts and seven inches," the clerk responds.

"Is that a record?"

"No, but I do all right."

We always enjoyed a bawdy laugh. I credit her with passing down to me my fun-loving disposition and crazy sense of humor. But most of the time our interactions were nowhere near pleasant, and they became more unpleasant as I gave up eating compulsively and moved toward a life far different from hers. Most of the time, any slight provocation moved us to screaming at each other.

But about what? Meaningless battles. A minor issue, with some slight nuance of misunderstanding, could send us raging into the night. Even in the good times, we were living in unrequited longing lament, wailing lyrics to songs like "Didn't We" sung by Thelma Houston or "Sometimes When We Touch" by Dan Hill. We were always a few beats off. Any lamenting about unrequited love, opportunities just missed, any country tune about good intentions gone awry, or anything that wailed of endless longing was our painful mantra. And the way we hid from that longing was by fighting or eating.

Relatives report that even though my mother thought I was an adorable baby, she left me all day in dirty diapers. She always complained of "extreme tiredness." She kept her own body filthy, and mine too. It kept others away, out of our lair. She wanted us together at home in the kitchen. Making my way out into the world, I incurred her wrath. "Sure people like you. You're clever. You've got them fooled. They don't know you like I do."

As I grew into adulthood, instead of crying with me about our separation difficulties, she would rant. In becoming a respected, thin professional person, I had forsaken my heritage, the East

Coast, and especially, her. I once took her to an Overeaters Anonymous (OA) meeting that a number of my former patients would attend. After the meeting, many members came up to her with "Wow, thanks for having such a great daughter. She really has helped me. I am so happy she's opening these clinics and offering such a service to the world. You must be very proud."

My mother stepped back and shot me a dagger-look and replied, "Yeah, she thinks she's hot shit sometimes."

My patients backed away in stunned disbelief.

In fact, my mom inspired disbelief in many who met her. The first night she met Yves, she stayed up late in our kitchen banging cupboards, slamming skillets while frying eggs, and screaming about something I'd said or done during the afternoon.

"What do you think of my mother?" I asked sheepishly, waiting for his refined European interpretation.

Responding with his rather formal, English-as-a-second-language propriety, he ventured, "Well, she's a bit uncivilized."

She appeared uncivilized to most people, messy and smelly. Best description: she lived as a bag lady with a roof over her head. In eating, hygiene, or decorum, she was utterly savage. Any thought that came to her mind immediately flew out from her lips.

I loved and hated her.

As her obesity spiraled into more self-abuse with prescription drugs, I learned exquisite footwork dancing around taking care of her, worrying about her, or waiting for her to blow up about something. Whenever I felt a brief reprieve, especially when we'd had a good time together, I'd get blindsided out of my reverie. She'd ruminate, work herself up into a lather, and then attack. "You'll never be any damned good, you ungrateful piece of shit. You're just like your father. You don't care about anybody but yourself."

Then the fights would start, beatings accompanied by accusations of evil intent. I gradually learned not to fight back, not to defend, and not even to care.

I'm not sure whether my intermittent attempts to treat her sweetly were motivated by actual love or by my desire to appear to be a "good daughter." I wanted to escape the *bad seed* feeling. I do recall feeling true love and compassion on the afternoon we went to see Broadway's *Kiss of the Spider Woman,* starring Chita Rivera.

We'd waited in the line for half-price seats, which turned out to be all the way upstairs in the last row of the balcony. By the time she got up all those stairs, huffing and puffing and sweating, her aroma preceded the mounds of shopping bags she was toting.

We made our way past a long row of young, starched-collared men already seated for the matinee. As we jostled our way in, I saw them making faces, laughing, and looking disgusted. They were doing exactly what I had always done. In that instant, however, I did not join them as judge and critic.

I was the daughter.

I wanted to punch them out and scream, "Yeah, she's smelly and unkempt, but *stop*! This is my mother. This is my *only* mother. She may be disgusting to you, but she's my family. Stop making fun of her."

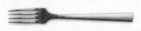

I feel a tear getting ready to drop while I remember that painful moment. I am brought back by Leon as he urges me to answer him. I have apparently been staring straight through him for a number of minutes. I resent him for bringing up my mom. My teeth are clenched. *Her energy doesn't belong here. I can't let all of that in while at such a peaceful place like this.* Compartmentalizing my spirituality to retreat settings allows me to get "good" there and continue with dishonesty in my real world. Here I can live like a transcendent, better-than-normal person, avoiding all the painful, messy, dirty stuff. Real life can wait.

Leon and I join all the introductory trainees assembled to receive work assignments. Reverend Kincaid announces in a voice that seems harsher than I remembered, "Every trainee will work *zafus*."

We will spend the whole weekend stuffing the round meditation pillows.

Apparently Reverend Kincaid senses that his tone is harsh, so he reverts back to his customary melodic explanation. "We here at the abbey are all excited that The Bodhi Tree bookstore in Los Angeles has just placed a large order for these cushions. We are on deadline and need to get many out quickly." Perhaps my karma has moved up a few notches. I am now brought in from the wild to work on objects nearer to humans, albeit their tail ends.

Reporting for work, I know immediately I don't like this assignment. As usual, it's the *people.* There are sixteen of us at various stages of this project. I want to be alone or preferably with just one other person with whom I can keep up a competitive edge. I don't play well with others.

There are feathers and dust everywhere. Our white surgical masks don't help. Instead of my treasured outdoor, lonely construction outpost, I am assigned a work detail cramped in a small room, totally enmeshed with other people, and due to get feathered, if not tarred as well.

Maybe I can plead allergies.

I quickly see a way out. There is one job that is separated and away from most of the padding and feathers. The "finisher" at the end of the assembly line picks lint and dirt off the outsides and vacuums into the folds and crevices to render the pillows cleaned and black as coal.

No one else sees what I see. They are all relegated to being one of the pack, standing in the endless procession of pillows, stuffing and hacking. But I, a cut above, deserve to be a singular, solitary loner, a breed apart. I grab the vacuum as mine!

At the abbey less than twenty-four hours, and I am already accumulating great gobs of negative karma. First, I pull this vacuum trick.

Then, at the end of our first work period, I find myself trapped in a stairwell with a young, ponytailed blonde named Tiffany. I'm cramped and claustrophobic and want out. I gesture and grimace and smile manipulatively, trying to silently communicate that I want her to move aside. She is oblivious. When she isn't quick enough for me, I "tsk-tsk" and grit my teeth.

"Well, I guess you can't let me out, then?" I say, glaring in her face.

As she offers some lame excuse, I don't miss the opportunity to silently express my irritation.

I am a great tsk-tsker. I rarely pass up the opportunity to let others know my irritation and impatience. It comes out often with clerks on interminable telephone calls. When I am in this haughty bitch phase, people are too slow, too soft-spoken, too indirect and manipulative, too muckin' fuch. They all have the terrible "toos." I am constantly sent such "intolerable" people so that I can continually relearn life lessons about intolerance and impatience. These people are my teachers. As I can't stand *them,* I am compelled to learn new responses to old stimuli. And I know I'll soon be apologizing for my attitude.

Who wants to apologize all day long?

Painfully aware that I am acting like a "bee-otch," I can't stop myself.

Washing up for the education class, I hope to get a hold of myself. After all, how many apologies can one woman make? A favorite twelve-step phrase is: "If you meet more than three assholes in a day, *you* must be one of them."

But Tiffany was so unconscious of blocking my way. Doesn't she need to learn about herself? Isn't it my job to teach her?

Reverend Marianne begins the class as if reading my thoughts. "Be careful of your judgments, for they all come home to roost."

Mine rest quite comfortably on my hips!

She continues, "When growth is our goal, we become more open and available to feedback from our fellows. From this stance, we are a much more vulnerable target, less defended when painful barbs come our way. Enlightened beings might not ever read instructions on how to control the world. They might instead welcome the pains of *not* getting what they want. Their perspective would be more toward learning life lessons. The positive aspect to this is that spiritual beings live a truer, more organically correct existence. We are more open to all life experiences, and that includes the painful as well as the joyous. A sense of humor to accompany the broadened perspective certainly helps.

"There is danger in really seeking an enlightened view of one's life. For some it may be easier to lie back and pretend they don't see what they see or know what they know. Sometimes it is easier to remain unconscious. More enlightened beings need to be more careful. If you truly know what you are doing, the karmic consequences could be worse. Once you know, *you know!*"

"Well, that's not fair," I quickly blurt out. "If you know more and see more, you're punished more?"

If more conscious, am I guiltier?

I feel as if she is reading my thoughts as she continues. "In Buddhism, ignorance is accounted for. It is understood that you can't possibly know all the forces you set in motion with your actions. Therefore, you are given a little leeway and grace based on your intentions. Intentions count, but competing, winning, overpowering all have a price."

I speak up. "Well, that doesn't sit right at all. I'm a psychologist. We write volumes teaching people more effective ways to manipulate and control their environments so they won't hurt. We show our patients and readers how to practice certain assertive techniques in order to win results or ward off pain."

Still sounding demure, with a lilting voice, all sweetness and light, she eviscerates all self-help literature. "In the Buddhist tradition, training and enlightenment might initially have opposite goals in mind. In order to grow and learn, we need to experience fewer wins and a great deal more losses.

"The more enlightened you are, the more quickly you may reap more direct karma."

Boy, maybe I didn't really learn anything by grabbing the vacuum or forcing Tiffany to stand aside.

Don't I always seem to learn and grow more when things don't *go my way?*

Who needs growth, anyway?

And immediate karma? Aren't my problems with food my karmic consequences? Sometimes the feedback is immediate, but I just can't see it. Whenever I choose to eat instead of feel, karma shows up in my obsessional relationship with food. Later those consequences are graphically recorded by the numbers on the scale. When I behave out of sync with my own true Buddha nature, I will eat inappropriately.

THREE
No Free Lunch

At our next class session, Reverend Marianne cautions, "You also have to be careful of too much certainty. If you feel too secure in your position and resolve, you court disaster. You have to look for the subtleties. If you teach someone something that allows him to do harm, you are responsible. There is no escape from staying awake and aware. If you compliment the good works of someone to someone else who you know is jealous of the first person, then you are guilty of bad speech."

Well, talk about being damned if you do and damned if you don't!

I want to yell out, "Oh, for crying out loud! Enough already!" Instead, I sit quietly.

She reassures us. "Even so, don't be afraid to act or to ask. As long as we stay teachable and trainable, we probably won't stray too far from the path.

"Even when we make mistakes, the law of karma is compassionate. It exists to help us learn. We will see that the results we set in motion are consequences of our behavior. It is not a moral issue, but more like a natural law, like gravity. If you set certain energy in motion, there will be effects. As you live consequences, as you stay teachable, you'll get clues as to what behaviors you'd like to change. The more enlightened you become, the more quickly you can see karma working in your life. It's all teaching. It's all practice."

I'm gradually surmising a downside to all this. Once you know, you can't pretend you don't. Your inner spirit won't let you. When you stay awake, you know. From time to time you can overeat to dull that awareness, you can act a little unconscious, playing a little dumb, but, whether you like it or not, *you know*.

There is a Sufi story about an elderly king preparing to die who was indecisive about which of his three sons deserved his fortune. He called them together, proposing a test he'd use to measure their merit.

"You must kill a chicken without being found out. If anyone knows of your deed, it will not count."

His eldest son went out to the edge of town and slaughtered a chicken behind a tree. He returned to his father's court, triumphantly waving the dead carcass, bragging that he'd killed the chicken without being found out. A villager piped up from the crowd, "I was out hunting in the forest and saw you kill the chicken." Case closed.

The second son went to a far-off lake, took a boat to its center, and killed a chicken before returning to his father's court. After his declaration, another villager piped up that he'd been out at the lake fishing and heard the chicken squawk and witnessed the act. Same verdict.

The third son, who was often considered the most sensitive and not as clever or smart as his brothers, then came raging up to the throne, eyes ablaze, clutching a squawking chicken under his arm. He bowed before his father and, with tear-stained cheeks, blurted out, "THE CHICKEN KNOWS!"

Your own chicken knows.

We're all accountable to self. It matters not what the world allows.

I guess I'm actually blessed with a metabolism that lets me get away with absolutely nothing.

With an extremely economic, efficient metabolism, everything is utilized, nothing passes through, and any excess shows up immediately. Now I learn it is not just metabolic, but my moral misdeeds can also result in gained weight. If I want to eat less, I have to stop living lies, face the truth, and admit my faults.

We all have an internal sensor—call it instinct—that lets us know if we are true or false. All our chickens know. There is no escape from truth.

We break class for lunch. Chairs are scarce and there's a mix-up with the seating arrangements in the dining hall. I think Roger is holding a chair out for me. "Can I take this?" I ask as I pull it out of his grasp. Quizzically, he looks away with "Well, sure." He saunters off as I bow to the last available space and sit down to eat. Later I realize that Roger's not working as server today.

I've taken his chair. I have just used a fellow trainee to get what I wanted. Oh well, it is an honest mistake. How was I to know?

Yeah, but what if I had been paying attention? What does my chicken say?

How is it that inattention always seems to net self-serving results?

My slight unconscious errors in judgment just happen to get me what I want, i.e., the chair. Rarely do I err in the direction of "doing for" the other guy and leaving my needs unmet. No wonder I am so judgmental, railing at other selfish manipulators. Who more skillful to see but me? I spot it, I got it. There are no mistakes or lies in Buddhism. We're always being fully who we are. Somewhat in contrition, at lunch I cut only half a quiche serving and pass when second helpings come around.

At the afternoon session, Reverend Kincaid begins his lecture with "Persistent effort should be your key to carrying these principles back to your daily affairs."

Ruth, a young Brillo-haired girl who's been giggling with me and making faces behind her protective mask on the stuffing job, jumps in. "I'm still not convinced that meditation is a good idea for me. You see, my meditation time is spent in 'monkey mind,' watching my head race around from thought to thought. I rarely reach the mindless states I'd anticipated. I'm still motivated, though, because I know that I am such a novice and wouldn't even know Nirvana if I sat in it."

He responds, "You could even give up on the idea of *understanding* it altogether. No one can explain what Nirvana is, only what it is *not*. The student can only interpret new information from the perspective of what he already knows. It is hard for a monkey that has been on land for its entire existence to describe the experience to the fish that has spent its whole life in water. The fish can only ask questions based on what it knows of an aquatic world. How do you describe a wholly new medium? It requires a cosmic shift of channels. Stay open and available to any interruptions or changes that come your way. It will be your flexibility and willingness to *let go* that will illuminate your path."

Then the Reverend starts into that gratitude thing. "All life deserves gratitude." I'd always hated that talk. At my first support group meeting in 1974, I was incensed at housewives smiling about how grateful they were, as I sat in the back of the room wearing my size-24 muumuu and flip-flops listening to the "Sarah Syrups" talk about gratitude. I wanted to yell out, "Sit down, you skinny bitches!" I bring my attention back to the present and focus on what the Reverend is saying.

"The Buddha exists in all things. Keys to your enlightenment are everywhere. Whatever work you need to do and whatever spiritual dilemmas might cloud your path, all are signposts for your next right step. They will all be sure to present themselves in the process of life itself."

I blurt out, totally out of context, "How do you know if you are doing *your* will or God's will?"

"For the Buddhist, we echo Carl Jung, asking you to discern your little 's' self from your big 'S' Self. The larger Self is, of course, your Buddha nature, your essential voice within."

"Can your little self sincerely delude you into acting according to its wishes instead of your higher Self's intentions?" I query.

"We recommend consulting with other like-minded souls for guidance and assurance," he answers.

Ah, and twelve-steppers advise consulting a sponsor. Everyone needs a mentor. We all need to stay teachable in "beginner's mind."

I want to impress Reverend Kincaid with a popular line from a twelve-step program: "An addict alone is in bad company." But I'm too engrossed in his explanations. I love his short summation of this dilemma.

"Actions of the little self often leave a vale of tears behind. When you are operating from big Self motives, some great events go unnoticed, even to you. But enlightened action is usually not accompanied by grand gestures. This does not mean there won't be dramatic moments, stresses in life, gut-wrenching catharsis.

We needn't fear loss of the drama. The enlightened being begins to see life itself as the thrill. It's all a question of attitude and surrender. One rides the ripples much as a surfer jumps into oncoming tide.

"Enlightened action evolves from meditating regularly. It is like a knife slowly slicing water. Enlightened action creates no wake."

FOUR

You Spot It,
You Got It

I recall my first immediate karmic event in 1983: Asked to speak at a self-help meeting, I first go to meet my friend, Karen, for dinner. We select a place in Westwood Village where parking spaces are at a premium. Rather than pay for parking, I circle the streets until I find a back alley where many other cars are parked. There is a NO PARKING sign on the opposite side of the alley, but I'm sure that's not related to my space. *Can I get by?* I pull in and hurry off to meet Karen. Something just doesn't seem right. That "getting by" feeling always portends ill.

And what were my intentions?

Getting away with something?

During dinner, I'm distracted, guilty, and worried.

Just a little parking space, for goodness' sake. What's the big deal?

I just can't pull off the same old stuff in the same old way any longer.

The night has just begun.

Running late, we head for the meeting in Karen's car. Since it appears that I've just gotten away with something, for my talk I decide to lecture everyone else. My topic is *those people* who create problems and chaos in their lives, expecting others to bail them out. My talk is full of judgments and irritability.

I rant on and on, especially adamant and perturbed about "anyone who expects *me* to help them when they create messes." I explain how I can't stand those people with entitlement issues who expect me to help. I talk about how difficult it is for me to say "no" when asked. Instead, I might go along, help out, and then seethe with resentment.

Buddhists would point out that letting others think you will gladly rescue them when you don't really want to might be classified as "selling the wine of delusion." You are pretending to go along when you really disagree. Twelve-steppers teach that fixing others' problems is depriving them of a growth opportunity.

The meeting begins at 8:00 p.m., and by 8:30 I am full-throttle into my tirade against "wimps" and "users." I'm feeling awfully good and especially self-righteous—lecturing, judging, criticizing, floating in my own wine of delusion.

When Karen drives me back to my parking alley, the pavement is deserted. No cars! Every previously parked car, including mine, has been removed.

What the . . .?

There is no sign at all that any cars have ever been there. Not even a friendly note about where the cars have gone.

In a panic, but trying to appear in control, I stop a police car in the middle of the street and ask politely, "When cars are towed from this area, where do they end up?"

Directions in hand, I sheepishly ask Karen to drive me a bit farther. I am caught creating and advancing the exact behaviors I just judged during my talk.

At the tow yard counter, a sullen, overweight woman with downward-curving metallic nails continues reading her book and mumbles, "The charge is $50 for both ticket and towing. No credit cards."

"But I have only credit cards."

"So," she sneers, "what do you want from me?"

Again, I need Karen.

Luckily, she has the bucks. After an hour-long wait with Karen by my side, my car is returned to me. All the while, feeling exceedingly guilty and excessively apologetic, I keep asking Karen to wait with me. She seems none the worse for wear, keeping up polite chitchat, intrigued with the workings of the tow yard.

Just for the hell of it, I ask the attendant to check the invoice to see what time the towing took place. It happened at 8:15 p.m. At the exact moment that I was preaching and judging, I was creating my own identical karmic consequences. Just like in comedy, timing is everything.

Wow, this kind of direct payback could get mighty dicey.

As I continue to pay attention, I often find that whatever I notice in the other person is something I do myself. If I didn't have my own acquaintance with the behavior—not just at the table, but in all areas of my life—then I wouldn't even see it in others. If I don't want to have a fluid body boundary, constantly gaining and losing weight, undulating between large and small, then I have to pay careful psychological attention. I have to discern when I feel my own boundaries are violated, as well as recognize when I overstep the boundaries into others' lives. Most overeaters can easily fit into the category of codependents. We are very "outer" directed, feeling others' pain even more than they do.

We also are terribly sensitized to any transgressions of our own boundaries. We often don't even feel it at the time. Eating helps us dull a pain that seems so inappropriate and inexplicable. We might find ourselves in a plate of pasta, eating over some minor violation that we smiled through at the time.

Jungian psychologists posit about "projections," the idea that we actually make up who we want people to be and what kinds of behaviors we think appropriate, and usually manufacture what we see in a situation. It takes paying careful attention to tease out what is true from what is personal fabrication. In any event, whatever we make up does become our reality anyway. It is usually much easier to notice others' violations of us in this way than to see our own overpowering of others. To help in teasing out best behavior, Buddhists would advise, "Right action creates no wake." A handy device for evaluating your own behavior is the "KNIT" test. Before acting, ask yourself the KNIT questions:

1. Is it **K**ind?

2. Is it **N**ecessary?

3. Does it bear **I**ntegrity with who you really are?

4. Is it **T**rue?

If you can't answer yes to at least three of the questions, then it is wise to delay the action. If that's impossible, prepare to accept the consequences.

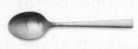

On the last day of the newcomer retreat, the monastery is celebrating with a festival for the great teacher Bodhidharma, a Buddhist monk who lived during the fifth and sixth century AD. We trainees participate with the monks in a highly ritualized celebration. We approach the altar in threes, bowing and dabbing incense on our foreheads.

It's all so pagan. I love it!

As monks drop lotus blossoms to the floor and we snake-dance around the altars, I catch my first glimpse of Reverend Kinnett, founder of the abbey. I had heard about her and read her books for months. Viewing her perched on high in the lap of the fifty-foot Buddha statue, I note her excessive weight, reminiscent of my most rotund self from years past. Her head is, of course, shaved, and highlights her face, which sort of resembles the pet English bulldog at her side. She silently exudes a certain reverence and respect for herself and all beings.

I find it pleasing to be in her presence, although I can't really tell why.

But as I look at her face, I immediately recount all the harm I have done in the past two days—grabbing the vacuum for myself, glaring at poor Tiffany in the stairwell, taking Roger's chair at lunch, and even almost swearing in a monk's lecture!

Does being in the presence of a spiritual being make people feel guilty? Do we recognize our own shortcomings more? Do guilty people strike out at whoever causes them to see themselves? Is this a key to most rage anywhere? Do I rage because I feel guilty, thus continually piling on more layers of guilt? Is that why so many people of faith are martyred and crucified? Is it because people don't want to look at themselves? If that's the case, then who wants to be spiritual? Even more so, who wants to be a therapist?

Does my mom feel guilty around me? I know there are a lot of clichés and jokes about Jewish mothers and guilt. I know Catholics lay claim to the same need for penance. Knowing I'm a stereotype doesn't quite help. Being a therapist—and a family therapist at that—makes it doubly worse.

I should know better. I should understand more. I should behave differently.

Oh, stop "shoulding" on me.

Could it be that I became a therapist, working continuously on myself, so that I could offer up better, seemingly plausible psychological defenses? Did I choose to be a therapist to avoid being crazy? I didn't want to be like my mother. I was great at psychoanalyzing her behavior. "You see, her condition is explained as *lacking in genuine empathy*. She had no ability to identify with any feelings from the other person's shoes. She wanted to love me, but she waged great internal battles that Thorazine and Elavil did not quiet. Just like a wounded animal, she couldn't empathize with her prey. If lions paid attention to the fact that the zebra or giraffe might be pregnant, they would never eat.

Just like when Hansel and Gretel venture away from home, the witch appears. My mom was angry that I had ventured out, creating a life full of valor. When I came home from play, the witch was inside the nest.

Mom just wasn't able to separate well. What mother really can? I wouldn't know. I never had children. I became a family therapist too early in life. Watching families struggle in painful recoveries, I saw that raising a family involved a lot more work than most people anticipated.

When people ask, "Why didn't you have children?" I quip dismissively, "Could never afford the therapy." Truth is I feared I might do to them what was done to me. Only later, when I dug deeper and closer to the bone, would I find that I also feared someone hating me as much as I hated my mother.

I am protected from the painful separation struggle by investing in my books, my readers, and my patients. Thus, though sometimes painful, the relationships are time-limited and I am mostly in control. I can maintain a professional distance. A caretaker has to be distanced enough to hold a steady hand to pull out that splinter without flinching too much in her own personal pain.

My mother didn't have that luxury of distance. When I was twenty-two and living in Greenwich Village, I picked her up to go shopping in the first new car I ever owned, a red Fiat. On the way home, she commented, "You seem down. What's wrong?"

I hated those times when she saw right through me. They led me into a false sense of security. Often I'd opened up, only later to be terribly sorry and badly burned. But this time, I forgot.

"Ma, I just had an abortion."

She fell into a scowling silence.

Cautiously expectant, I carried the groceries up three flights to her new Brooklyn apartment.

Following in distractedly, she left her front door ajar, and began a deep wailing. "I knew I never should have let you go away to college. You learned to live like a *shiksa* in those college dormitories, those *whore*houses," she screamed.

I started changing clothes to leave. She moaned and spewed, "Look what you've done to me. I can't believe what a no-good piece of shit you are. How could you do this to me? What will everyone say?"

At that point, "everyone" didn't know yet.

I begged, "Please stop screaming. I didn't do this to you. I did it to *me*. This is about ME! It's not about YOU."

"Shut the fuck up. Is this what you learned in college?"

She barged through the bedroom door, finding me in my slip. She walloped me in the head, and then chased me around the small apartment, punching and kicking.

As I ducked behind the French doors to the dining room, she came at me, so hysterical that she didn't think first, but instead bashed her fist into the glass, grabbed my hair, and pulled my head back through. A neighbor heard the glass shatter and rushed in to pull her off. Thank God she'd left the door open. As he pulled her back through the glass, cutting her upper arm, she glared at me and screamed, "Look what you've done to my arm."

It was always me.

Ignoring her own injury, she pushed the neighbor into the building hallway with me close behind. The door slammed and the bolt clicked. I cowered in my slip. Her neighbor looked horrified as he quietly returned to his own apartment.

I fell in a heap on the steps, sobbing. She left me there crying for three hours as neighbors, returning from work, stared quietly.

Many shook their heads. My mom was new to this building. No one knew me. They just left me sitting there. I couldn't go out on the street with no clothes. I cried and begged and eventually she let me in with nothing further said.

Years later, in a random conversation, Mom said something that made me wonder why she knew so much about abortions. I asked her point blank, "Mom, have you had an abortion?"

"Yeah, it was when we were newly married and your goddamn father was already starting his running around. We weren't sure we would stay together, so I went to Philly and got rid of the thing."

Compassionately silent, I sat in shock.

"Ah, it's a long time ago. I don't want to talk about it."

There it is. That's why she beat me up. My pain put her in touch with her own. Unable to feel it, certainly not able to share it, she did what she knew best—she attacked. If only I could have known of her pain at the time. If only we could have cried together. If only . . .

That memory brings me back to the abbey, where I've now been immersed in all this talk of compassion and caring. *I am starting to see more of the other person's argument. I'm walking a mile in Mom's shoes.*

I will eventually see how much of the spiritual journey has to do with forgiveness, for self as well as others.

Upon departure, carting my bag down to the gate, I'm startled as I meet up with Leon. I decide to do a living amends. I'll be nice to him to make up for my earlier coldness. Sometimes it is better to change behavior than to issue "hear ye, hear ye" proclamations about how badly we feel.

"How did you like your stay?" I ask.

"It was truly great for me. I got the same feeling here like I felt atop Machu Picchu in Peru. I am at peace, content, and in the presence of greatness. It's a cosmic homecoming."

I hold back from giving my lecture where I explain how Bill Wilson wrote a letter to Carl Jung asking for help for alcoholics. Jung responded that therapy could not help, because those with addiction suffered a spiritual malady, seeking *spirits* in the bottle. He felt that alcoholics and addicts were plagued with a "hole in the soul." Instead, I stand quietly in my own hole, but equally at peace.

FIVE
Stay Honest

Is life a crapshoot? Is compulsive eating the door prize? Is America's obesity epidemic a symbol of how we cash in the chips of excess? Why, in a nation of abundance and luxury, are so many of us starving and ravenous? Why is *more* rarely *enough*?

No matter how blessed with abundance, many of us still battle the "gimme more" monster to the ground. And it's not just *more* we want, but a devious, manipulative, and conning *more.* After a humongous binge, deciding to "get away with it one last time," we'll promise to totally fast, always playing catch-up ball, jumping on and off the scale. We want to see if we've beaten the odds. No matter what, most gamblers ultimately lose. And I don't mean weight.

How do compulsive shopping, gambling, and stealing relate to eating and purging? If you think about it, it's a logical progression. Those who eat to excess and then vomit for weight loss think they got away with something. They eat all they want and then get rid of the consequences. They defy the laws of karma for a while. When they first start out, they binge, but don't gain weight. Eventually, the vomiting stops working and they gain weight anyway. I've admitted many to treatment centers who were bingeing, vomiting, and crying, even while on Prozac and regaining weight. Their gambling days were over. All bets were off.

In many cases, when the vomiting stops, shoplifting starts. Repeatedly throughout my professional career, I had patients who stopped vomiting, but then became shoplifters. That is the time when each comes face-to-face with the "Gimme More" Monster. The "Gimme More" Monster often debuts in the lap of luxury and abundance. It doesn't matter how rich you are. Petty theft is a way to beat the odds, to reap ill-gotten gains. Haven't we been shocked by headlines of wealthy Hollywood stars caught stealing in expensive Beverly Hills shops? Do they *really* need to steal?

The grabber mentality—"Gimme More" Monster—does not die easily. I had certainly fed and nurtured my monster. I had no idea about the connection between overeating and dishonesty as my early teenage shoplifting developed into a well-honed art. Oddly, I would only lift things I could easily afford. I craved the sport, not the bounty. I once took my college roommate into a store, instructing her, "Don't take your eyes off me. I want you to tell me later how many items I've lifted."

"Thirteen!" she shouted boldly after we left the store, with a smirk on her face like "Gotcha this time."

"Twenty-eight." I smiled broadly, admiring my haul spread out on the park bench around the corner.

That career ended abruptly when, caught at a market with a T-bone in my jacket, I was gratefully relieved when the grocer warned, "We will let you go this time, but don't patronize our store again." I never did and I never stole again. Well . . . let's define *stealing.*

In 2003, through a bit of manipulation and cashing in on a favor from one of the owners, I called to see about staying at Oprah's favorite spa retreat—the Miraval Arizona Resort outside Tucson. It costs a minimum of $1,000 per night.

"Sure," chirped a secretary. "Bill would love to invite you for two free nights, which include a spa treatment each day. Enjoy your stay."

I clear my schedule and with bags packed, I prepare for pampering, spa cuisine, exercise classes, hiking in the desert, stretching, and yoga. Within a few hours I am roaming the exquisite desert-landscaped grounds and am promptly admitted to my plush accommodations. My hostess shows me around and points out each snack bar and café where healthy canapés are available twenty-four/seven and sugar-free cookies and ice creams are there for the asking. While explaining all the facilities and activities, she informs me, "Oprah and her friend Gayle were here all last week filming a special. The weather has now blossomed into spring, so you are privileged to come at an opportune time for our best weather and quieter schedule."

Ocotillo plants are just beginning to bud, showing their red conical flower clusters. Barrel cacti here are large and old, so they all lean to the south. Birds chirp continuously as little bunnies scamper behind desert shrubs and bushes. I feel my eyes glaze over as everything in these environs calls out beauty and serenity. I am totally stoked, blessed, and delighted.

My suite, from its entry foyer to its private terrace, exudes southwestern luxury. The down comforter stands at least a foot above the mattress, and there are overstuffed leather couches in front of the fireplace. I am content beyond my wildest dreams, just sitting and taking in the caring this place affords.

But not for long.

As I admire the bathroom facilities, I slather on some Cactus Cream Body Lotion, provided in a nice two-ounce bottle. I love it. It smells divine, like light cucumbers and maybe some sage. It seeps into my pores easily, immediately plumping up my skin.

I must have more of this.

I learn the lay of the land, traipsing from fitness center to dining room, from yoga center to lecture hall. My head lolls from side to side as I take in all the beauty and attention to detail the place affords. But I'm on a mission.

Cactus Cream calls. "Gimme More" rides high.

I eat my meals quietly and mindfully, ever grateful that I am totally alone to savor my own experience—commenting, exclaiming, or explaining to no one.

If only I had a little more Cactus Cream.

I am lusting after this body lotion.

I attend all the great lectures, fitness classes, and cooking demonstrations, and all the while Cactus Cream relentlessly beckons.

At the gift shop, I don't ask the price of the body lotion. I don't intend to *buy* it. I want to steal it. Even though my stay has been totally complimentary, I still want to push the edge and get away with something. I spend not one minute on gratitude for all that's offered. Instead, I plan to cheat, steal, and win more.

Here I am, treated like a lady and offered full service and amenities by friendly and not overly intrusive staff. Anything I want to eat and drink is at my disposal. They probably think I belong. I probably even pass for someone who could afford the place. Even though they can't do enough for you here, I begin plotting to get even more. I revert to street ways in a second. I operate from some inexplicable drive to beat and cheat the system.

It's not about wanting the cream. It's about beating the system and getting away with something. Isn't this what compulsive eating is all about? Isn't this why we jump on and off the scale all day? Can we beat the odds? As for all these niceties, I've always relished high class as well as low down. I enjoy every luxury hotel and meal hosted by TV shows and lecture organizers, but if the bill's on me, a clean bed and hot shower are usually quite enough.

Give me Gray's Papaya, the cheapest and best New York hot dog, or take me to Le Cirque. I like both, though Gray's is more physically filling while Le Cirque is more aesthetically pleasing. I can have a spa facial for $100 with a few cream samples thrown in, or feel equally pampered picking up an out-of-date Almay or L'Oréal cream from Odd Lots Liquidators. I like bargains and elegance, but favor neither.

In truth, though, I am most attached to the bargains. I like to cut a deal, cheat a little. This getting more for less is the same thinking at the heart of all the cheating on our diets. Whom do we cheat? What do we get away with? The chicken knows. He knows we're feeding that "Gimme More" Monster.

There is a continuing attraction to the excitement of the dark and dangerous, a strange juxtaposition between feeling overly entitled and nondeserving, between righteous indignation and "mea culpa." Twelve-steppers say, "We're egomaniacs with an inferiority complex." We're driven to do better, to crawl into the light, but at the same time scurry back under the rock.

I devise a plan to get my Cactus Cream. Just like visitors in third-world countries explain traveler's diarrhea with "It's in the water," I decide to get more than my share in the water *bottle*.

All staff at Miraval constantly promote drinking water. "Here's some bottled water if you'd like" seems to be the Miraval mantra. "Are you drinking enough water?" is asked by each fitness instructor before and after every class.

I'll empty those bottles, and then go around to various locales spritzing the lotion to fill up the bottles.

I may have to buy extra luggage.

The spa locker rooms have the most lotion. With three or four stations of mirrors, including wash-up counters, makeup centers, hair-dry alcoves, ear-cleaning stations, magnified eyebrow-pluck desks, and any other grooming activity a lady might enjoy in front of a mirror, there's room aplenty for me to squish out my prize. Each station has a large bottle of Cactus Cream with a pump.

I decide the ladies' room in the fitness center is probably the best opportunity. Few people use the facilities, as most go to their own rooms for showers. So, those bottles are full and they get little traffic. It is ideal for my plunging and plundering plans.

After dawdling at the mirrors waiting for three latrine users to finish, I find myself totally alone. Time to get started. I get off about ten or twelve good squishes and then someone comes in. I stealthily set the bottle down in my complimentary Miraval canvas sack while smiling at my intruder, who goes into the nearest stall. She comes out much too quickly and smiles. I'm sure she thinks I'm normal.

Quickly, a spark of sanity returns. For some reason, I gain a moment of perspective: *What a genius—spending time at Miraval beating the system for a few ounces of lotion. What are you doing? Are you nuts? Are you seriously considering spending your time at this luscious resort seeing how you can steal, yes, steal, extra body lotion? Can you not afford to buy a bottle in the gift shop? Do you not have thousands of bottles of excellent body lotions at home and access to a super-saver deluxe, extra-ounces, "derma-friendly" brand from the 99¢ Only Store whenever you run out? What is going on?*

Ask the "Gimme More" Monster.

This monster appears wherever and whenever I least expect it, catching me totally off guard, screaming, "More. Mine. I deserve special treatment according to my own rules. I want to get away with something."

It's the same voice that shouts out from the all-you-can-eat buffets and drive-thrus and clearance racks in clothing stores. She's a gluttonous monster that never gets enough and thus keeps me feeling like I am not enough. She's the same voice yelling for her own room at Shasta Abbey. There's no advance warning or prescriptive preventive plan for when she'll rear her greedy head.

What stops me? What brings that moment of clarity? What creates the reprieve? Am I accessing my Buddha nature? Is this who shows up when I gain the wherewithal to stop a binge in the middle of a bag of trail mix or leave a dessert midplate or put back the pile of clothes I'm preparing to charge? Such devious excesses are clearly linked to self-destruction, offering punishment much more than nurturance.

Such punishments, like overeating, are a subtle form of gambling. When I roll the dice and gorge down mass quantities, I later lay odds on crash diets and quick fixes, hoping to suffer no consequences. Am I escaping karma? I believe a decision to binge is definitely a lapse into compulsive gambling.

In more than thirty years of quelling overeating, I can tell you that the monster continually morphs into stranger styles and personae. Sometimes I see her and can head her off. I typically recognize her when halfway through excesses. Sometimes a phone call to a similarly afflicted friend will help. Then I can immediately stop and turn around. The monster never dies, but accessing my personal Buddha nature allows me to catch it faster and change direction sooner.

In the midst of my squishing Cactus Cream into water bottles, clarity and determination wash over me. I reach into my canvas Miraval bag, pull out my half-full bottle, and smooth the entire contents over my legs, arms, and chest. *I'll use what I can at Miraval and take nothing illegal home.* I quickly toss the bottle in the trash.

I think it's over. I think I've stopped.

Oddly enough, the spa portions at lunch seem more than enough.

SIX
Give Up to Get

Getting truly honest may entail loss. If I honestly and carefully examine my eating, I'll find I can surely get by with much less food. I'll surely take in less. If I look carefully into my closets, I'll find I can never mix and match enough outfits to use all those clothes and costume jewelry necklaces. Eventually, I might even move to freely and lovingly giving things away. These spiritual concepts creep slowly inside my skin. Planted while I'm on a national book tour, they fully bloom in department stores around the country. Remember my first abbey entrance wearing too much fragrance? Oddly enough, my first major encounter with the concept of "giving up to get" is staged over perfume counters. Giving away to get results is "losing to win."

It is 1994, and *Fat & Furious,* my mother-daughter book, has just come out. Right before my scheduled presentation at an international conference for food media writers at the Drake Hotel, in the heart of Chicago's shopping paradise, I leave at the lunch break to find every department store on Michigan Avenue running some kind of PWP or GWP.

Every cosmetic company worth its lanolin offers periodic deals for potential customers to try its products. It's either a GWP (**G**ift **W**ith **P**urchase), which means you buy something and they give you a gift, or PWP (**P**urchase **W**ith **P**urchase), meaning you can get a lovely tote full of goodies after you spend a minimum amount on other products. You've probably seen some form of black bag hanging from the sleek shoulders of highly styled Lancôme women. This particular summer, Clinique featured the yellow canvas and Estée Lauder had a summery blue stripe.

I spend half my life playing at makeup counters, taking advice from women sporting five shades of eye shadow. I also absorb skin care tips from those decades younger, already genetically predisposed to glowing, turgid cheeks. Knowing it's a scam— the cheapest stuff is just as good but without the expensive packaging and advertising—I still struggle to leave these counters reserving my rent money but maximizing my freebie possibilities.

So, on a cold February afternoon I saunter out onto Michigan Avenue and stroll into Bloomingdale's, where I nab an excellent PWP travel kit of Perry Ellis 360. I'm sidetracked from my mission to pick up a sample of Clarins's new eye gel at Neiman's. On the way, I sniff a glorious, sweet fragrance. I amble around in a trance and make my way over to the counter for a sample spritz.

Vowing en route that *it's probably way too expensive, I can get it from my knockoff guy in Manhattan, and I'm not going to buy any,* I'm greeted by a gorgeous, long-legged, big-haired lady. "Do you know that Angel's heavy, sweet smell is made with no flowers, just vanilla, chocolate, and patchouli?"

"Do I know? This afternoon I'm giving a lecture about eating disorders. I certainly know from vanilla and chocolate."

What's not to like?

"Do you know about Angel's special travel package?"

I let her show me the nice black suede goody pouch, filled with a purse-size spray, body lotion, soap, and travel towelettes, all for $75. Not yet allowing myself that lay-down-star bottle, I figure I can spring for the travel pack.

I can give the lotion to my friend Monica for her birthday. I'll just keep the purse spray, soap, and towelettes for myself.

Big Hair clinches the sale with "As a Christmas in June special, this offer allows you to get your travel bottle refilled totally free of charge all during the month of June."

Ka-ching, ka-ching, I quickly calculate. Charting my travel plans, I figure I'll use up the purse spray by May to be ready for a summer fill-up. This is such a deal.

It's destined, meant to be.

Having it shipped saves me sales tax, and I head back to my conference feeling quite satisfied even though I've had no lunch. Shopping for bargains is one of the best ways to avoid overeating, but it brings on an addictive euphoria that can be costly.

Throughout the spring I enjoy and use up my little spray bottle. I am now ready for the June refill. Ever mindful of what is most important—getting mine—I pack up the empty Angel bottle to refill while on tour for the paperback release of *Fat & Furious.*

Since this bottle has run low, I also take along a few sample bottles of my usual and customary Jessica McClintock perfume. No kitchen flavors here; it's light, airy, and floral. I'm pretty safe wearing it for any occasion and with any outfit.

Starting the tour in New York, I decide to get my Angel refill at Saks. I struggle through their makeup department, a world-renowned shopper's gauntlet. You can't get through the aisles without being attacked by aggressive sprayers and hawkers, luring innocents to their counters with "Want a facial?" "Need a makeover?" "Smell this." "Look here."

I find them to be quite snooty and synthetic with their puffed lips and tattooed brows.

Such competition in the beauty aisles could make one ugly.

I stroll up to the Angel counter where I am greeted by Daryl, who is standing next to a gigantic pumping machine. My pulse races as I pull out my bottle with "Fill 'er up!" Daryl smiles sweetly but apologetically, explaining that the machine's nozzle doesn't fit small travel bottles.

"The refill offer applies only to the bigger bottles. If you'd like instead, you can buy a special-deal $90 bottle. It holds more than the $125 bottle and comes with a small funnel for fill-ups."

Another damn special promotion.

My lower lip quivers. I stammer, trying to complain, "Well . . . well . . . well . . . the woman in Chicago knew what size she was selling. I guess she really wanted to make the sale and didn't really care about me."

"I do apologize for her mistake," he sing-songs in that corporate, "no one is really responsible, but we're all terminally guilty and don't give a shit" way. He hands me a similar sample purse spray of Angel as a bit of amends.

"Maybe some other stores have a way to fill up your bottle," he consoles in a haughty tone, indicating it would only be a *lesser* store than Saks.

Satisfied that I've at least gotten a new purse spray out of the deal, I thank him, shrug, and head uptown to Bloomingdale's.

Pay attention. I am now one sample ahead. I don't get what I expect, but I still *get*.

Heading north, I reach into my purse for my tiny Jessica sample bottle and dab some behind my ears. I'm accepting that Angel will no doubt be scarce. The Chinese cabbie asks in heavily accented English, "What is you puhfoom? You smell so goooood."

I tell him the name, but it's difficult for him to pronounce.

"Jussssssigggaaaaaa?" he struggles. It's clear he wants to get some for his wife.

"Expensive?" he asks.

I can't resist. I have to give it to him. I know I have at least one other Jessica sample in my luggage. I just don't know if I have enough to last the whole tour.

I reach into my purse. "Here. Give it to your wife, please. "

Delighted, he thanks me profusely.

I'm now up one Angel, down one Jessica.

The next day I check into my Philadelphia hotel where the desk clerk inhales deeply and asks, "What is that lovely fragrance you're wearing?"

"Jessica," I answer, feeling strangely caught up in some weird, perfumed Rod Serling *Twilight Zone* episode.

I wonder if anyone is secretly filming the scene.

I had found two more Jessica samples in my luggage, so upon hurried checkout (I'm scheduled for a TV interview), I hand him the small bottle with "Here, hope your girlfriend likes it."

He beams.

This is turning into a lot of fun. I'm in the middle of promoting a valuable book about food abuse and traveling the land spritzing, like Judi Perfumeseed.

After the TV show, my escort whisks me to the train to head south to D.C. I ask if we can stop by Saks Fifth Avenue to get the Angel refilled. She's up for it. Again, the Angel representative had no nozzle small enough for my sample bottle, but she hands me two samples for my troubles. Note: I am now up three Angels, having given away two Jessicas.

This letting go is really working.

That afternoon I arrive in Baltimore to have steamed crabs with my friend, Joel. I promptly tell him my perfume saga. Before I finish, the waitress appears and approaches me dead-on with "Is that Jessica you're wearing? I just adore that perfume, but it's too expensive for me."

I'm on the floor.

I know now that I have to give her my last Jessica sample. But I need to have some Jessica. Angel might be too sweet for some of the venues I'm working. Even though I don't really want to buy a full-size bottle to schlep for the rest of the trip, I have to let my sample go.

Oh well.

I hand her my last sample with "Here, you've got to take this. I can't explain, but I have to give it away."

She beams.

By now I'm quite intrigued by this perfumed dance. So I ask Joel to take me to a nearby Saks to check out the Angel possibilities. The woman behind the counter never heard of the "Christmas in June" promotion, but she gives me a handsome Angel travel sack, with nothing inside.

I still have to replenish my Jessica, as I feel Angel is too sweet for book signings. Joel and I race through the mall to Macy's, where, lo and behold, they're having a promotion at the Jessica counter. I tell the saleslady my weird story. She is so intrigued as I buy a full bottle of Jessica along with a free lotion that she throws in with three small sample bottles and an extra soap.

Now I am back to my original three sample bottles and I am ahead one Jessica soap, three Angel samples, and an empty Angel carry sack. This starts to sound like a Christmas jingle of some kind.

I'm content. All's well with the world.

To take the story full circle, when I return to New York I head back to Saks to tell the tale. Daryl leans in furtively and whispers, "What the hell. If you don't tell anyone, we can use our tester filler and fill up your little sample bottle."

Wouldn't you?

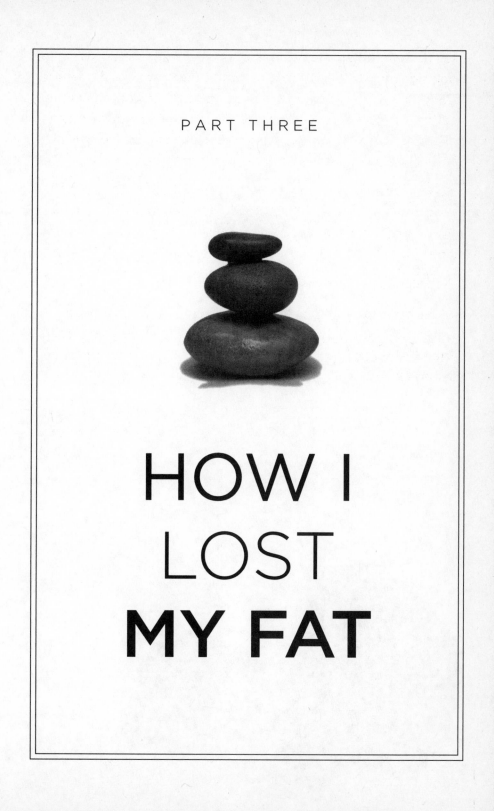

PART THREE

HOW I
LOST
MY FAT

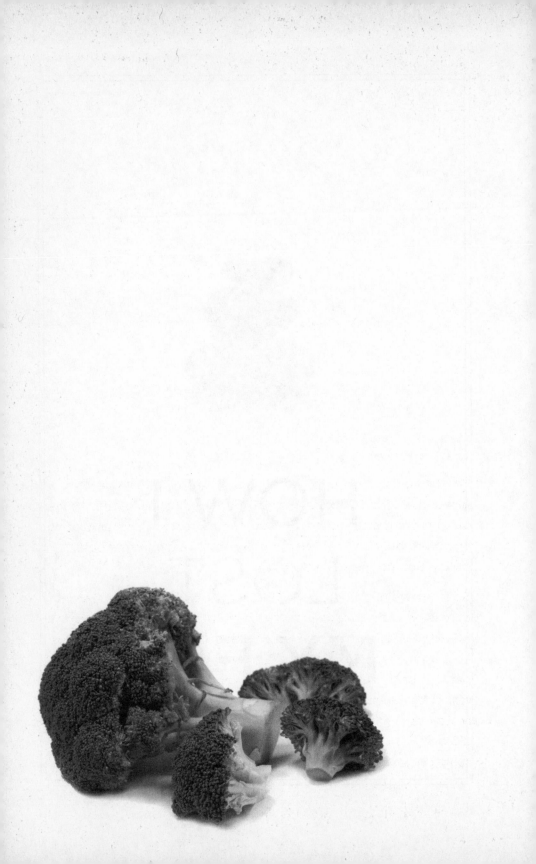

ONE The Body Doesn't Lie

I am obviously becoming more and more uncomfortable with dishonest behavior while liking the lightness of giving up. As I let go of more material objects, I am not interested in accumulating any more guilt and self-loathing. Honesty becomes my best policy. Something is shifting.

So is my weight. In the early 1990s, my perimenopausal weight comes on with a vengeance. I'm living mostly by Denise Austin's 80-20 rule, though mine is 95-5. Ninety-five percent of the time, I eat and exercise in a weight-loss or maintenance mode. Then, 5 percent of the time, I eat more or exercise less. The scale never responds accordingly. I can eat sanely for weeks on end, and no matter how much I pray to break 150 pounds, I hover at about 153 or 154. I lust after 149 so that the black bar on the doctor's scale doesn't have to move over a notch. I want to jump on in front of the nurse assistant and move the bar to only 100. I so want to think of myself as a "normal" person. Sometimes it seems like I get away with things. Despite my "hovering weight," I can eat a lot at the sushi buffet or too much sugar at a party, and the next day I find my weight down to 151. I am so tired of trying to figure it all out, examining what exactly I'm "eating over" and addressing those "fear of success, Jewish guilt, codependency" issues. After half a century, I grow tired of body image and weight loss as the major topics of my life.

But I'm destined to lose even more.

On a bright, sunny morning, Yves joins his motorcycle club for breakfast and then a ride through the Angeles National Forest. As he makes a left turn, an older couple pulls out from the side of the road and crashes into him, and in an instant takes his life and many of my dreams.

Dear, sweet Yves had been with me every step of the way. He had been there for all the lawyer meetings, all the endless repairs of our facilities and vehicles, taping all my lectures, sharing all the dinners as we discussed our "baby," the treatment centers. It consumed us; but, like all couples who run a business together, we found a way to survive. He'd really been the wind beneath my wings.

Without him, I no longer have the same enthusiasm to show up at HOPE House. I don't even care about it. I stop noticing the details. I become willing to let it sink or swim through the efforts of those I had put in charge. Though still there to advise and encourage, I have no energy for *fixing* anything. I no longer care to convince all those television viewers and seminar participants about the true nature of food obsession. When I started my first treatment center, I got a lot of flak for some of my ideas, and I found the debate stimulating and energizing as I confronted resistance. But after Yves' death, I gave up all the fight.

My whole life was developing addiction treatment programs. When my favorite aunt Hope was dying of lung cancer, I told her, "I'll name a daughter after you."

"Well, get married first," she said with a smile. Thus, HOPE House (Helping Overeaters through People & Education) was born. Now that it functioned and could operate without me, I was willing to walk away.

I didn't just stop monitoring; I stopped worrying. It would be someone else's job. Maybe no "worry" was necessary, but it was clear I could no longer play the part. Meditation made that seat too uncomfortable; it no longer fit.

The great dream of glitter and glitz on television also took on a different hue as I got to know more about it. *Maybe we avoid intimacy so that we don't see beyond the rose-colored glasses.* I took some of the patients on the shows with me. This sometimes required extra counseling so they weren't consumed with fear before or afterward. Despite being fearful, most were eager to show themselves.

At the same time, many of the talk show hosts were bored and disinterested. I guess they had seen an endless array of shrink after shrink bringing on suffering souls splaying their lives straight to the camera. I started having bad feelings about my involvement with this medium. Although much in love with the "entertainment" aspect of television, I felt awkward parading people's tragic diseases. When so much intimacy is paraded so blatantly, everyone is cheapened. When a person casually names him- or herself an "incest survivor," no one comprehends or attends to the horror that is truly involved.

And then there were (and still are) the shows that turned human pain into three-ring circuses, appealing to the lowest human denominator. Real-life stories were made cheap. It seemed such a violation to reduce profound issues down to catchy sound bites condensed to six-minute segments between commercials.

But I continued, and as a result more treatment centers were opened based on our model. Membership in Overeaters Anonymous grew. It was a privilege to get the word out. There were situations where significant changes were possible. On one *Maury Povich Show* we did an intervention with a single mother, her teenage daughter, and a sweet, beautiful eight-year-old, all of whom were very overweight.

Maury agreed to pay all the expenses of treatment for this family. Our policy stated that we would not treat a child without his or her parent. Mother and daughter were flown out to Los Angeles, and we admitted them to HOPE House. Within twenty-four hours they left, AMA (Against Medical Advice). The mother stormed out of our facility despite the generous gift of full treatment and all expenses paid. What caused her to bolt? Just a simple thing like food? She had expressed interest in losing her own excess weight while she was on the show; however, once in treatment, she balked at being required to eat in a weight-loss manner. We required that every resident eat on a low-carbohydrate, high-fiber food plan. But, as often happens, she expected the total focus to be on her "problem daughter." She didn't realize that the whole family system would need to undergo change. She just didn't want to actively share in her daughter's life or to pay careful attention to her own eating. She would have none of it. If she couldn't freely eat whatever and whenever she liked, she'd pack up her daughter and leave. At the time, I felt such sadness for this poor young girl, and still, these many years later, wonder what happened to her.

So there were joyous as well as heartbreaking aspects to the media blitz. I knew that anyone in my field would have welcomed and been terribly grateful for the opportunities afforded me, but instead I withdrew. I became chagrined that so many were content with the medical model of seeking the great God—*diagnosis.* It seemed that once proper labeling was found, then everyone was content. People wanted to know what slogan to wear on their T-shirts. "I'm a codependent, compulsive eater, alcoholic, adult child, woman who loves too much." Just knowing the label is only the beginning. There is so much work after that, and so much surrender. Most shows didn't have time for that messy, undefined, "wait and see, stop and listen" kind of talk. Though I grew increasingly uncomfortable, the shows kept asking me back.

Unfortunately, I was already gone. During more than one TV taping, I found myself glancing at my watch, praying for the segment to end. I was seeking a deeper level of involvement. Divining diagnostic categories and sending people to twelve-step groups just wasn't going far enough. Labeling people as sick is a fundamental *first* step and gets their attention, but developing new ways to live and new values to live by is even more necessary. Few wanted to hear about all the work involved, and I had grown tired of carrying the message.

Actually, I had no choice in the matter. As I told Shinzen, I was clearly too uncomfortable to continue. I seemed to be racing cataclysmically to remove myself from the spotlight faster than anyone can chant *nam myoho renge kyo.*

Following up on Leon's suggestive nudge at the abbey, I decide to get away to something totally alien. I sign up for a tour trekking the Amazon jungle. This tour is filled with herbologists on an international mission to save great stores of rain forest medicines from destruction. I'm also on a mission to try to get over losing Yves. Later, I'll find that it's a journey toward some of my Jewish roots and into my vital, vibrant body.

There are no roads leading into Iquitos, so our tour's propeller plane lands in the last settled outpost at the edge of the jungle. After a four-hour motorboat ride away from all civilization, we arrive upriver at the base camp nestled beside the Amazon River.

We machete our way through jungle growth each day and listen with rapt attention to herbologists and anthropologists as they teach us about the local flora and fauna. Nights are for bat watching. Sometimes we awaken before daybreak to paddle out onto the river and watch the sunrise. I'm half-awake, crouched low in a dugout canoe, ignoring the birds, but loving the stillness and dampness of the morning dew.

Despite the early hour, birders are full of enthusiasm to spot rare species. A big guy named Carl, who wears all the right gear, yells out something like "yellow-bellied sapsucker." Twenty-four birder eyes dart to the sky following the turn of Carl's head. They all spot the dot. Then, notebooks and pencils are seized, proper notations are made, and I hear a victorious sigh with each new entry.

I wish those birders could keep quiet.

At the end of our weeklong trek we're invited to walk across "the canopy," a rope ladder one hundred feet above the jungle floor. The tour guides assure us we'll be safely harnessed.

Even so, that means if we do fall, we'll end up slammed into a tree. I decide to follow Vern, who gave himself the ladder walk as a present for his seventy-second birthday.

If Vern is in, then I sure as hell have to try.

With no conscious thought or fear, I quickly volunteer.

I want to feel empowered again, want out of my painful mourning treadmill.

At daybreak, we head out for the canopy walk. After extensive training in how to hook and unhook our harnesses, how to rappel down a tree without looking at the ground, and how to say a few "Hail Marys," we are ready to roll.

Before I have time to think about what all this training really means, I am standing atop a hundred-foot tree. Two large ropes are stretched parallel to each other and the ground. These ropes extend from my tree to another tree two hundred feet away. At intervals along these two ropes, three-foot loops are tied to ladders suspended horizontally above the ground. The rungs of the ladders are the "walkway." The two larger ropes are the handrails.

Yikes!

Each time I place a foot on one rung or a hand on one space of rope, a counterbalance takes place somewhere else. In this precarious situation, I sway every step of the way.

This "canopy walk" requires intense concentration.

I'm up for it. After all, I've been intensely focused on meditating.

I'll take it one rung at a time.

I won't look down.

Focus on feet.

Stepping cautiously while keeping my eyes on my feet at all times, I don't realize how scared I am. As sweat pours off my face, I watch the racing droplets rapidly disappear into the lush foliage below. I look past my feet only once, staying focused on toes.

I feel a strange connection between my pounding heart and racing breaths and the screeching jungle creatures. My heart sounds out the same staccato cadence. We're all in this together. I feel such faith in myself and the universe. Dripping with sweat, walking up in the treetops, I feel a tremendous "yes" to the jungle and to my life.

Finally reaching the last ladder rung, I see a four-foot space of nothingness extending over to the anchoring tree. Our instructions are "jump quickly, hit the tree, rappel down."

Stay focused.

Swing.

Made it to the tree. Great! Didn't smash too hard.

Now, push off. Let out a little rope.

Some more.

Now again.

And again.

Within a few minutes, I'm safely back on terra firma and extremely grateful.

I am so connected to my lean-machine, jungle-creature, purring, prancing body. She channels something strong and powerful from somewhere far beyond her own skin. Her heart pumps electrons out to a rain forest that is alternately approaching and avoiding, welcoming and repelling, birthing and decaying.

My lean machine morphs into a sleek black panther. Instead of a roar or growl, I seem to purr quietly to all the animals in the jungle, "I can do anything!"

And I know I can.

I keep vibrating for the rest of the day and late into the night. I feel so calm, so centered, and so confident. Feeling pumped up on adrenaline alternates with a strange quiet and calm. I sense a definite connection between taking risks, focusing on the body, and landing firmly in the now. Where else can anyone be? I fall asleep to the same jungle sounds I'd heard during the entire trek, and know with every fiber of my being that this time I'm a part of it all. I sleep deeply and completely at peace.

A week later, I land in Cuzco.

This charming colonial city, high in the Andes, remains quaint and unchanged from its earliest settlement. Most tourists and spiritual seekers head directly to Machu Picchu, either by train or bus, bypassing this old town.

When we arrive, the hotel staff instructs us to drink a cup of coca tea, made from coca leaves, and then take an immediate nap. They assure us that thus fortified, we'll have no altitude sickness. I am eager to drink the tea and have my nap, as an altitude headache is already throbbing. We'll soon learn that those of us who follow the advice do great, and those who don't are sick for three days.

After the nap, we board a bus that takes us to some ancient Inca shrines. I don't expect much. I've read Shirley MacLaine. I know where the best spiritual hits really are.

Machu Picchu is the place for spirit. Nothing will happen for us in this town.

Instead, I'm on my way to getting zapped, although I'm unaware of it at the time. And by a sexy woman, no less. The shrine's name is *Sacsayhuamán* (also known as Saksaq Waman), pronounced "sexy woman." Since I'm working on my third book, *Hot & Heavy,* about the connection between eating and sexuality, the irony isn't wasted.

Our guide explains the history of the place, how no one knows how short, ancient Inca peoples carted these 300-ton rocks up the mountain. And why here?

After climbing seventy-five feet up and surveying the top of the structure, I notice many two-inch-wide canals carved into the stones. In ancient times, the canals held water used by priests in ceremonies that welcomed young boys into manhood.

Hmmm. And the name of the place is pronounced "sexy woman."

Our guide instructs us to stand in the center of the labyrinth and speak our own name. When the Incan priests entered that indentation, their voices reverberated and echoed a thousandfold. Our Peruvian guide invites us to "see if you might be a priest as well."

I watch as, one by one, my fellow travelers try to hear their own echoes by speaking softly on this hallowed ground. Each gets no sound whatsoever in return. They ask the guide why he's making such a big deal about hearing an echo.

Then it's my turn. I move in rather nonchalantly, expecting the same. I step up, planting myself squarely on the sacred spot, and whisper softly. Immediately, my voice echoes across the canyon. Some kind of vibration moves through me—like a large gong that has just been rung. Reverberations ripple around my stomach like a stone skipping across a lake. I feel my whole body resonate like a steeple bell. I close my eyes and feel my blood pulsate against artery walls. I can hear the ringing of my voice over and over again. My feet feel stapled to the ground as I sway in one spot.

I have found home. I'm vibrating and swaying; I'm blissful and content. I am completely connected to my body and focused in the here and now. Just as I felt when I was atop the jungle canopy, I'm both *in* and *out of* my body at the same time. I'm home. As an army brat, I was a nomad, always reinventing myself at each new location. I never felt at home. I never even knew what home should feel like. But this is it—I finally know what home is.

As I pivot around this circle in the setting sun, I sense this place knows me and I know it.

I know I have to stay on this mountain, at this shrine, listening for more. Forget the tour bus. Forget the other scheduled sights.

I beg our leader to leave me. "You can pick me up on the way back into town."

He reluctantly agrees.

For the rest of the afternoon I play like a child on this mountain. I can't leave my new home. I sit a while meditating, and then casually stroll around watching a family picking dandelions for dinner. A flute player strolls by; the echo of the flute's melody is pure and enchanting. He plays on, circles me, and then leaves as quietly as he'd appeared.

Then, an older man comes by and leans against the rocks and watches me. For some inexplicable reason, I go over to him. From within the folds of his clothing, he draws out a flat leather pouch that he unfolds to reveal a number of crystal stones. He urges me to take one.

"I am shaman. You are priestess, a medicine woman," he states matter-of-factly.

This marks the first time I'm called that.

I don't question a thing.

Where is my doubting Tomasina?

"Must show you the ritual, how to pray at this site," he offers.

He takes my hand and leads me back over to that central spot where I felt those vibrations. He demonstrates, raising and lowering outstretched arms à la Superman. Lying fully prone with arms outstretched, he rises again to standing, then bends over, then stretches his arms skyward.

I follow his directions, mimicking his moves, similar to the sun salutation pose in yoga or the prostrations monks perform at Shasta Abbey. Drawing hands up in front of his face, he bows *gassho* and in an instant is gone.

Then the bus arrives to pick me up, and I'm gone too.

On the ride back to the hotel, I ponder the day's events. *I don't understand why I feel such a strong body/spirit connection in an Inca shrine atop a mountain in Peru.*

Why here?

Why now?

What connection could I possibly have to this place?

The next day's trek up to the summit of Machu Picchu, often referred to as "Lost City of the Incas," offers great exercise and neat anthropological finds, but leaves me cold. The site does nothing for me. Clearly, I'm not buying what others have to say about this land and these people.

But why had I vibrated so at a lesser-known shrine? What do these Incas have to do with me?

Possible answers emerge as we travel back through Cuzco and down again to the Amazon River. Before getting back on the riverboat, we have an afternoon's break to hike around Iquitos. This small town lies four degrees south of the equator and is inaccessible by land. Modern tourists fly in, but for centuries it could only be reached by river.

I decide to walk around and explore. In the center of town, I look up to a landing above a tailor shop. Almost destroyed by the jungle elements, but faintly visible to my squinting eyes, is an etching of "Goldberg & Sons" chiseled into the stone facing. Below it is a Star of David.

Strange.

Had I come to a South American jungle town to connect with some kind of Judaism? Is this my promised land? Why does my body pulsate near Inca ruins?

I'd later learn that there had been and still remains a significant settlement of Jews in that tiny, unpaved jungle town. They'd initially come in the middle of the nineteenth century from Europe and Morocco as entrepreneurs and adventurers to gain fortune from the rubber trade. Most were young and single. They married native women, forming a very interesting *mestizo* or hybrid culture.

In his book about descendants of these people, *Jews of the Amazon: Self-Exile in Earthly Paradise,* Ariel Segal notes that these adventurers "found lust and got lost." They lost their self-conscious Jewishness.

Well, I'm also a wanderer/nomad type, endlessly recreating myself. I bet some of my ancestors were up atop those rocks at *Sacsayhuamán.*

At age ten, I'd had my first experience of self-conscious Jewishness. My teacher in the small schoolhouse in Lebanon, Missouri, loved me, and even let me play Santa Claus in the Christmas play. The following September I approached her, as instructed, with "I will be absent Monday because of the Jewish holidays."

She backed away. Staring at me as if horns had sprouted, she whispered softly, "I've never seen a *Jew* before."

I had no idea what was so strange about us or why she was backing away. She used to like me. What went wrong? I felt exactly the same as a minute before, but she changed noticeably toward me from that moment on. I was now altered in her eyes. I wasn't just fat. I was Jewish, too. After that first childhood experience of prejudice, most such encounters later in life would be more subtle and sophisticated.

In Peru, European settlers had found a way to assimilate, but still hold onto themselves as well. That kind of synthesis is exactly what I was after. I didn't want to be a Buddhist, Christian, Muslim, Hindu, or Jain. I just wanted to find my personal "Judi-ism."

Right here in the Amazon was definitely a piece of it. These settlers developed an all-accepting form of spirituality combining Judaism, Christianity, and jungle myth. In his investigations, Segal found the same people attending Friday night Shabbat services and then going to Catholic mass on Sunday. During Segal's visit, an aged congregant died requesting interment in the Jewish cemetery following a Catholic high mass.

Now this kind of assimilation appeals to me!

These people combined Jewish history and jungle mysticism, performing many Machiguenga tribal rituals using the Star of David to ward off the jungle's evil eye. A fascinating blending of religion and superstition.

One sunny morning, a jungle shaman warned Segal he'd have showers by afternoon. Despite all his belief in Western science, Segal took his umbrella.

I, too, could choose to trust the jungle or fight it.

I could choose to trust my body or fight it.

It would all coalesce with what the body would allow. After all, I truly only extend to the boundaries of my own skin. When the body stops, the entire story stops. I'd just need to trust the wisdom of my organism.

A lot of this *mestizo* mixed-race history had to do with macho men and sexy women. *This certainly speaks to my ancestry. I could do this.* Little Incas hooked up with swarthy Mediterranean types to produce this vibrant, sensual spirituality.

I'd been zapped at sexy woman.

Did I need any more signs? *Maybe I'd had some ancestors who were adventurers in Peru. Funny, they didn't look Jewish.*

In his book *The Storyteller,* Peruvian author and Nobel Prize laureate Mario Vargas Llosa tells a haunting tale. A young, extremely intelligent Eastern European Jew with shocking red hair and a red birthmark covering half his face is constantly outcast and taunted in his native land.

I relate to the redhead's life because my life mimics his.

My fat is my birthmark. Growing up, I was taunted with this rhyme:

> "Fatty, fatty, two-by-four
>
> Can't get through the bathroom door.
>
> So she did it on the floor,
>
> Licked it up and did some more!"

In Llosa's story, the European redhead mysteriously disappears. Years later, his friend passes an antique store and in the window sees a picture of an Amazon tribe. Strangely, the tribe's witch doctor has the same red birthmark. In the picture, he is surrounded by tribesmen who seem to respect and venerate him.

Examining the picture more closely, he discovers that the witch doctor is his long-lost European friend! The former freak found home. He is vibrant, respected, safe, and accepted. In his assimilation, he combines Jewish angst and Indian cosmology. He lives in a jungle where humans respect all nature and thus other humans as well. They believe each animal has been transformed by the spirits into every other animal.

Buddhist reincarnation, perhaps?

We are all one and in it together?

Discrimination is ridiculous. As American society still finds "You big fat _____" the expletive of choice in most schoolyards, and judging the body of another is still perfectly acceptable, it would make sense that I would be trying to find a way to honor my body sensations and incorporate spiritual teachings.

I'd read Women Who Run with the Wolves. *I live near the Mojave Desert. Surely I can find a more convenient transcendence closer to home. There are Native American tribes in my own backyard that might have a clue to accessing the spirit through the body and the earth.*

TWO
Funky Body Booty

After I have returned from Peru, the Amazon woman within me blossoms. There is no keeping me locked down in hospital wards or private consultation rooms. As hormones rage with a last gasp before menopause, my spirit searches for more resonance in my sexy female body. My itchy feet will lead me to grovel in the dirt of New Mexico, enduring extreme heat and exhaustion to transcend my animal nature, and bliss on out to spirit. *What keeps driving me? I keep listening to my body because all my life's work and entire personal journey have been about helping me and others own that body—that funky female body.* I want to regain my Amazon experience to again feel that spiritual connection transiting through my body to channel that sexy woman.

Even though I'd initially found the connection at Sacsayhuamán in Peru, where I purred contentedly with all the jungle animals, I know Spirit lives for me in the desert. When I hike in the desert I morph into a lizard, basking in the searing heat. I suffer and survive! Whatever creatures and plants stay alive in the desert— they are the real survivors. We really demonstrate a will to live.

L'chaim! L'chaim! To life!

Maybe suffering extreme heat in a sweat lodge could help. It all sounds great in theory. But so far, each time I've tried a "sweat," I've run out on myself and the goddesses.

A new opportunity emerges as I just happen to be booked into Santa Fe. After delivering a great speech at the upscale and pricey La Fonda Hotel, I wander up Canyon Road, past all the elegant art galleries, into the raucous local hangout, El Farol. I've heard about their great tapas.

Happy to wear my new chamois suede skirt from a thrift shop in Chelsea, along with long, feather earrings from the street fair in Palm Springs, I look hot and funky. I wear not one ounce of that tourist turquoise sold in the plaza.

I'm a local.

At the bar, a slim man, dressed totally in that black, Santa Fe cowboy-with-a-bolo thing, tries to pick me up. He comes on with the usual "Show you the sights, li'l lady?"

"You know, I'm not the bimbette my outfit might indicate," I tell him. "I'm looking to experience more of the authentic Native American tribal culture. I'd love to find a sweat lodge."

He changes tactics and begins to listen.

Somehow I sense he's not the showy cowboy he appears either, so I explain my quest.

"In all my previous sweats I've left at first flap. I got out as soon as I could. I just couldn't stand it. I couldn't stand the heat. I couldn't stand the prayers. And, quite frankly, I really couldn't stand the people."

"Where did you do those sweats? California?" he asks with a condescending smirk. Most locals are down on Californians who have sold large houses for great fortunes and have now invaded the quiet hills of New Mexico, driving land values through the roof. They call it "Californication."

"Well, yeah," I respond. "They were in nice enough settings, one along Pacific Coast Highway in the hills overlooking Malibu and some down by Laguna. Very nice. It's never been the place that bothered me. It just didn't feel right to me. I always left at first flap."

"Couldn't take it, huh?" He again smirks at my efforts. I begin to feel like I am once again auditioning to prove my sincerity.

I rise to the bait. "Something about the whole thing didn't sit well in my body."

"Ha!" he chuckles back.

I continue with my theories about why it might be different for me this time. "Those sweats were all led by Westerners, male Westerners; nice people all, but men, and Western men. They seemed to be trying to act like Native Americans. To me it seemed they fashioned their speech to be slow and sing-song, affecting a Native speech pattern. They pretended English wasn't their native tongue. It all felt too phony-baloney."

I continue explaining to the cowboy more than he wants to know. "I'd love to find an authentic sweat led by a Native woman."

As he discerns I am not a player, but perhaps a legitimate *seeker*, he responds. "Well honey, we have 'the gathering,' going on all weekend on the outskirts of town. Grandmother Little Moon from Taos sometimes does sweats for women only. You just have to head out past Chimayo and then you'll find it."

With a dismissive hand wave, he offers up vague directions and turns away.

Somehow I know I'll find the way. This is New Mexico, after all. This is the "Land of Enchantment."

I know about the shrine of Chimayo, often called the southwestern Lourdes. In its low-ceilinged back room hang crutches left by cripples who exit walking. Stories abound of the blind seeing and the deaf hearing after they visit.

If it's near Chimayo, there must be healing there.

Finding "the gathering" is a cinch. Despite the cowboy's vague directions, I just follow the road out of town, and without effort, park my compact rental car next to a lineup of four-wheel-drive trucks and campers. People are milling around, speaking in low tones, being generally quiet and respectful. I fall in line, following others toward a distant drumming over a hill.

I'm reminded of the long walk down farmer Max Yasgur's path at Woodstock decades earlier. Then, as now, lines of us walked quietly. I follow the faint music, ambling toward a last glimmer of daylight.

Instead of the nude bathers and random guitar strummers at Woodstock, this Chimayo path is lined with stalls displaying beaded jewelry created by the Natives, a number of newly cured animal skins, and countless smoking cauldrons spitting out fry bread, sort of an Indian donut. Children munch these ravenously, ready to join the next generation of diabetics. So much is made of the alcoholism problem among Native Americans, but rarely mentioned is their rampant obesity.

But let's not digress. I'm off duty here.

A beautiful young woman with long, shiny, black hair approaches me knowingly. "Are you looking for the women's sweat?"

Not at all stunned by her picking me out, I answer, "Yes."

Maybe the cowboy had wired ahead? Maybe in the woods people just know stuff?

She leads me to a large, oddly configured tent. Ropes extend between two trees, and heavy woolen blankets are piled each over the other in many, many layers. A light-blue plastic tarp covers it all.

"I'm Marissa. I'm not a Native American, but my husband Luke has been following the Native ways for many years. I'm into beading," she offers, holding up her current project, a headband made of turquoise and white beads with little red dots. Picking up a smoking pail from the campfire, she swishes it up and down before her body, letting the sweet smell of sage waft up into her face. Turning around, she invites me wordlessly to fan the smoke up and down her back. She then does the same for me.

As I deeply inhale the burning sage, Marissa explains, "We are being smudged to smoke away any impurities. We want to be totally clean for our prayers and rebirth in the sweat lodge."

Smudging done, I settle onto the warm, dusty ground, taking in the woods and the fire. Tall, muscular, and very blond, husband Luke approaches.

Marissa beams, clearly proud of her handsome partner, while I marvel at the knee-high chamois moccasins worn by both of them. They are a light yellow-tan and soft like butter.

Luke explains, "I cured these deerskins myself. I have the last of 'em with me. They're for sale."

Well, now we're talking.

He further hawks his wares. "I can give you the address of a lady in Salt Lake City who makes up the moccasins. You send her the skins along with a tracing of your foot and she'll make you a pair."

Done deal.

After our transaction, Luke leaves for the men's tent and Marissa takes me to meet Grandmother Little Moon.

She's a very fat woman who gives me the once-over, and then nods a welcome.

"What are you doing here?" she asks.

Uh-oh. If she knows who I am and all I know, she'll want to pick my brain to help her with her eating problem.

Cautiously, I explain to her, "I am working on a book about women and power and what that has to do with overeating."

Nonplussed, she responds, "I am Lakota. Lakota respect women. In Lakota sweats it is okay for a woman to be on her moon."

Evidently this is a very big issue. In other tribes, menstruating women are not allowed into a sweat lodge. Explanations about this aren't all that clear, but the general prevailing wisdom is that "women on their moon" are just too spiritually connected.

In fact, some tribes send menstruating women to live in a tent away from the general encampment. They are to rest and commune with the earth while other women care for their children and husband. The flowing woman is to relax and meditate and listen to Mother Earth. She is invited to come back from these outings as a shaman to tell the elders what she has learned.

In other tribes, women are banned from some lodges. It is feared that they are such spiritual conductors that they might take all of Mother Earth's energy and leave none for anyone else. Their menstruating status is a gifted privilege rather than a diagnosis or the "curse" we bear in more "modern" cultures.

I repeat to Grandma Little Moon my historical drama. "I've been in at least six other sweats where I ran away. I don't know why I keep coming back."

She just smiles.

"You can keep a bathing suit on under a T-shirt or just go naked."

I'll have suit and shirt, thank you very much.

Grandma Little Moon beckons me to crawl into the tent. Marissa and some other young women have already entered.

"I'll be finishing up some prayers around the campfire, praying to the four directions, spreading tobacco, and smudging any latecomers. I'll be in later," she says.

Later? How much later? How long do I have to sit and wait in the dark and heat?

I'm already calculating.

If she's not coming in until "later," whatever that means, then those in early will have all that extra time with the heat, legs cramping, enduring, and waiting.

I see that others are lining up to hunker down and crawl through the flap. I saunter to the end of the line. As each woman enters, she crawls around the fire pit, taking the next available spot on the other side of the tent. Grandma Little Moon's place is reserved on the right-hand side of the entry. I manage to be the last one in. So I'm on the left, next to the flap, opposite Grandma Little Moon, and closest to the escape route.

She crawls in soon after me, settles herself, and starts beating her drum. Quietly, just under the pounding tone of the drum, she announces ominously, "If anyone has come here for entertainment, you may *become* it."

I immediately assume the warning is for me. She then tells us that our *fire keeper* will be a man; she's okayed it. Evidently there might have been some question of female energy being contaminated by a male getting near the sacred rocks. He'll be responsible for staying outside at the campfire, keeping the rocks hot, and shoveling in new ones each time we open the flap. He'll follow her orders. Maybe his being in a servile role makes it okay.

She closes the flap and with no warning plunges us into immediate pitch-black darkness. The only sound is from her pounding drum and my heart revving up. She chants and offers up songs. The rest of us huddle quietly in the darkness.

I rock with the beat of the drum, getting into swaying with the rhythm of her chants. The heat's rising, though. I have difficulty making out her directions. I'm feeling a bit of panic.

Beginning to freak, I get distracted from myself briefly as Grandma Little Moon explains, "The first round of prayers is for ancestors, the next is for children, then for family, and then, by fourth round, for all Mother Earth's creatures."

I've never been able to understand this love-of-all-the-creatures thing.

"We will open the flap between each round. At that time, anyone who wishes can leave. We'll begin with ancestors, and starting on my right, go around and each offer up a prayer."

Oh my God! There are twelve of us in here. The more people, the longer it takes between flaps.

If we have slow talkers, it could get really heated up before we even open the first flap!

I pay no attention to any of their prayers, as I am busy praying for my own survival. The heat isn't bothering me. It's the closeness, the lack of air.

My ancestor's prayer expresses gratitude to Grandpa Stockman for escaping the pogroms, immigrating to this country, and giving me such a great life.

I'm even more grateful when the flap opens. I gasp, gulping in the coldness, as I am right near the door. Grandmother tells us we can raise the tent portion behind where we each sit. My blanket goes up instantly, rushing in more blessed cold air. I crouch down like a panting dog, butt high, and gulp.

Soon it is time to close the flap and let down the raised blankets. Grandmother asks if anyone wants to leave.

This is my moment.

This is where I'd always left. There's nothing wrong with leaving. No shame. No foul. No one cares. I'd just sit outside and wait for them all to finish without me.

That's what I'd always done.

Instead, I take a deep breath, exhale fully, and proudly say nothing.

I'm staying past first flap!

While the flap is still open, our male assistant takes a pitchfork and shovels in six more hot lava rocks, the flap slams shut, and we are again submerged into total blackness. Then, it gets much hotter, much faster. Now it's not the lack of air. It *is* the heat. There's always something.

I remember a psychic once telling me I'd been forged into strong steel by a very hot, incendiary past. "Your mother loved you enough to take on the dark side, carrying negative energy so that you could work through your karma and lead others into the light." Somehow thinking about heat forging steel calms me down.

Little is visible in the soft glow from the rocks. I make out a few figures, but mostly listen to voices with no clue of the source. There is chanting going on, and Grandmother Little Moon periodically gives instructions. Then, following to her right, each person in turn has something to say. Some go on endlessly, often about alcoholism in their families. I make out the low mumblings of a thin young girl who says she is offering up prayers for her brother. It really sounds like she's taking the opportunity to vent her frustration at his continual drunkenness. She goes on and on about what he does and how helpless she feels.

I don't hear any further prayers or chants, not even my own. I am so hot and cramped and doggedly focused on survival. I'm having a really hard time of it.

I surmised earlier that most of the women in the tent are younger than I, and slightly more eccentric. I figure that's why they keep chanting loudly with no apparent distress. I don't know the chants, and wouldn't have the breath to chant them anyway.

When it comes around to my turn to offer up prayers, I say something short and sweet. I'm into conserving energy. I'm too hot as it is. Then I notice an aged Native woman beside me. Though she'd been right ahead of me, I hadn't seen her when we all filed in. She leans close and looks at me knowingly.

I don't say a thing as I gaze back. We sit that way for what seems like twelve hours. Then, watching my continual body shifting while beads of sweat pour off, she speaks softly"If you lie down, it gets easier."

She must know what I'm going through.

Lie down? Why not?

Isn't that the message throughout this entire journey?

At each juncture, I am tested, need help, and follow suggestions. I lie down.

I stretch out on my side, feeling the coldness of the earth caress my cheek while I huddle up, fetuslike, placing my right hand back by my butt.

With half my front on the cold ground, panic dissipates. I don't hear any more prayers and really don't care. I'm loving the immediate relief. A gentle rain has started outside, and perhaps that is cooling us down. It just doesn't seem as hot as it was before. Somehow, I manage to stay for all four flaps.

Maybe it's the cooler, rainy night. Maybe as I'm getting more into this, I'm able to stand the heat. Maybe I've spiritually transcended my body. Our leader is a Native. We're women only, and well-versed women at that. Also, the older lady is helpful and supportive, offering me a plan for survival rather than encouraging suffering to achieve some kind of goal. This is not a macho-male, endurance-dude thing, but a letting-go, melt-with-the-flow, Delicious Doll thing. I surrender and stop fighting. Could it be bearable because I've surrendered?

Who cares? I stay.

No one is suggesting I endure and ignore my distress. Rather, the suggestion is to do what you can to flow with things. Be pragmatic and get the job done. For me, this is all so authentic, appropriate, and organically correct. My truth-seeker, supersensitive self is not at all put off, finding nothing abrasive, disjointed, or out of sync. My judge is asleep, having pounded her last gavel—for now.

I don't remember the drive back to Santa Fe. My body cleansed, maybe more grounded in earth, I relish my new sense of well-being. Somehow I feel like I am more *in my body,* and thus genuinely in my life. Instead of an enemy to be kept in check, my body has become a vehicle for transformation. I know there is more to learn about a body-spirit connection. I've just been with women who seem to know all about this. And guess what? I enjoyed getting funky, muddy, and sweaty. And I relished not being the teacher, not leading. I was content to listen and learn.

But those teachings and that experience become incorporated into my retreats and seminars, as I change more to an "allowing" rather than dictating style. For the next few years, in my retreats, I offer sweat lodges in Palm Springs, all run by Lakota women. So many of my participants needed that surrender when they found their edge of resistance. All were allowed and encouraged to trust their bodies and leave when things got too uncomfortable.

In ensuing years, keeping up a hectic, bicoastal lifestyle and still traveling with lecture gigs becomes more of a burden. Whenever problems arise, I tend to call Taos and seek telephone guidance from Grandmother Little Moon. I complain about a fixed menu of problems, but mostly some form of the big two: romance or finance. She offers gentle guidance and calm reassurance, inevitably suggesting that I sit quietly and listen to my body.

Meditation? Paying attention? It's the same old song.

The body doesn't lie.

Be still and know that I am.

I know the body is the key to my salvation.

When I allow time to meditate, with or without yoga, I again feel that pure resonance and vibration. I can even achieve it sitting in a subway, configuring my body into the straight-back, hands-cupped, Zen-tripod position. That position transports me back to mountaintops in California or Peru, the tent in New Mexico, or hikes in Palm Springs. I am sexy woman; Native-American-deerskin-moccasin woman; Machiguenga Amazon tribal woman, all knowing, all peaceful, pure and simple.

The yearly phone calls to Taos continue until just before September 11, when I am living uptown from "ground zero." I call Grandmother Little Moon even though I don't have a specific complaint. I have what some twelve-steppers refer to as the "**R**estless, **I**rritable, and **D**iscontents." Gotta RID myself of these feelings.

My major dilemma continues as usual: What do I want to be when I grow up? Do I want to continue on the lecture circuit, advising and training? Or do I want to stay still and listen? I complain to Grandmother Little Moon of skirmishes with lawyers, agents, seminar planners, TV producers, publicists, insurance companies, web hosts, and neighbors.

Grandmother Little Moon responds to none of this. Her voice has a deeper, more serious tone.

"You are a medicine woman. All medicine women are calling me right now."

There's that medicine woman thing again. How do they decide someone is a medicine woman?

"There is great medicine coming. You are being made strong to lead the rest. You are being prepared first. Something is coming. You will lead."

She doesn't bother to ask if I want the job. She assumes I've been gifted and will rise to the occasion. Instead my little 's' self starts her rant.

"But I don't wanna!"

I've never wanted this. I'm not cut out to be a leader. I want a house in Scarsdale with 2.5 children, a woody station wagon, cute tennis outfit, and a standing weekly manicure appointment. I don't want to lead. I don't want to be prepared. I'll take the end of the line, thanks.

With no inkling as to what could possibly be in store, I decide it's time to bail.

What can this Native woman know?

I've found many surrogate mothers in women like Grandmother Little Moon. *But how do I connect with women closer to my everyday existence, closer to home?*

THREE

Crack an Egg

Soon after Grandmother Little Moon's 2001 instructions, I continue a heady personal debate. It's between my introverted self who wants to be home reading and my extroverted self who loves the psychic, almost sexual experience of connecting with large audiences. I still want it all. I'm totally ambivalent. My extrovert is morphing into an introvert. My panther wants to roar like a turtle. For me, I can always tell when I'm lying because my eating tends to become excessive. I am slowly gaining weight and need to get away again to sort things out.

When I consult with Shinzen, we decide that another stay at the abbey might help. As I call up to register for the *Jukai* retreat where many devotees will be taking Buddhist vows, Reverend Kincaid explains that I can just listen and won't have to take any vows. He also has a surprise for me. "This retreat marks the opening of our new guest house. Each trainee has a private room and separate bath and closet."

What? No hondo? *No floor? No tiny cubicle for my clothes?*

"No way!" I blurt out, before taking any time to think.

"I want to sleep in the *hondo*. I want to sleep closer to the monks. I don't want to change a thing. Somehow, that feels more like the abbey to me. It reminds me of my first defiance and surrender. It allows me to give up a little."

"Okay, there will be ten overflow-ers in the *hondo*. You can be one of them."

Maybe I'll even take my own zafu *just in case I choose to sit for a few sessions on the floor.*

No way! What am I thinking? I'll stake out a bench space and leave it at that.

Boy, this letting go sure takes a lot of holding on.

I make sure to offer some kind of food commitment to my mentor before leaving. First things first. I call her and report, "I'll take no second helpings unless the first portion allowed is too small for a normal meal. If that's so, then at the next pass of the bowls, I'll take another spoonful. I'll eat in a somewhat-meager-to-moderate fashion. I'll take some packets of artificial sweetener for morning coffee, eat bread as served, but limit butter and other fats."

Pay attention. Calorie quiz to follow.

After my food is in order, my mentor asks, "What do you think you want to get out of the week?"

What kind of a question is that? What do I know?

I start feebly with "My attraction to the monastic experience resembles my early 'approach-avoidance' love affair with twelve-step programs. Even with major criticisms of the style and manner, I yearn for that overriding sense of peace and tranquility."

In truth, this was a Buddha call. I was becoming more and more attracted to gentle people, quiet ways, and peace. At my seminars and retreats, I was teaching mindful eating techniques like at the abbey, and I was starting to walk more gently on the planet. These monks, so diverse, with such varied pasts, living in harmony and peace, are definitely my kind of people—seekers and questioners, ever searching. They know there is *more* going on.

"I want to look at adult decisions I might have handled differently. I want to continually acknowledge my part in contributing to how my life unfolds. I'd like to feel better about how things went with my mother. I've been so busy defending against the guilt trips she laid on me that I've avoided facing the truth—that I'd been mean to her sometimes. I feel badly about that."

We make amends when we don't like who *we've* become.

"I also want to learn how to pray."

In my head rumbles a deep voice from a 1950s radio show quoting Alfred, Lord Tennyson: "More things are wrought by prayer than this world dreams of."

Applying reinforced silk wrap and crazy glue to my nails, and then painting them a muted beige, I make an appointment for a retouch the day I get back from the abbey. With all that in place, I start packing for an even colder stay. It's December. As I assemble long silk underwear, boots, gloves, hat, and scarves, I find that the same suede fur-lined jacket I took on my first trip is still the least offensive.

Why not? Those who were previously offended can reopen their wounds, and I'll have a whole new crowd to appall.

Let's not forget they wear shoes made of leather.

I will need sweaters and warmer gear, so once again I battle with the plethora of bright colors and dramatic statements. The multicolored, plaid acrylic sweater I ordered from a catalog will have to stay behind. It's not that warm anyway. Luckily, I have an old fisherman's knit from Goodwill. *Surely Buddhist types will appreciate such an old classic.*

Actually my closet has changed since I started my explorations into Buddhism. There are many more neutral colors, beige predominantly, and I'm developing a classier act. I often tell friends, "Think pearls, ladies." I enjoy the statement of making no statement. My garb is following my psychic changes.

I pack with great enthusiasm as I look forward to another week away. I'm fairly sure they won't brainwash me or totally change my whole life. I may also find answers about this public speaking thing. The enforced meditation might help me to make a more consistent effort when I get back.

I manage to read the "*Jukai* Retreat" directions on the flight up and realize there was some reading homework. *Oh well, I'll read what I can on the plane and trust my novice "beginner's mind" to cement in any loose edges.*

I sure hope they appreciate that even with bulky sweaters and boots, I've managed to whittle all of my belongings down to one fairly medium suitcase.

Reverend Kincaid giggles slightly as he greets me at the front gate. "Well, you requested sleeping in the *hondo,* so we've granted your wish."

He's distracted and busy with all of the lay trainees arriving at once—all needing special room assignments and tours of the new guesthouse.

"Judi, will you be able to get yourself settled in? You sort of know the layout down there. After you get organized, take a reading period, and then next on your schedule is meditation at 5:30."

He's treating me like an old-timer.

I smile and bow profusely, dragging my bag down the hill to "ye olde" luggage room.

Maybe I've made a mistake with the sleeping arrangement. It would be so nice to have a closet.

Getting to the bathhouse early, I grab one of the primo cubbies near the door. I stake out a large expanse of towel rack for my beach-sized, albeit now more subdued, flamingo towel. My competitive race for creature comforts has sadly begun.

I lithely trek up to my graveyard to read before meditation. A spring warmth brings the fragrance of pine needles to my eager nostrils. *How great to get away from the city.* The snow peaks are still here, as well as the small volcanic mound beside them. My graveyard is just as I'd left it. I bow to all the shrines and then settle in to my reading of the *Kyojukaimon* and the Buddhist precepts:

1. Cease from evil.

2. Do only good.

3. Do good for others.

4. Do not kill.

5. Do not steal.

6. Do not covet.

7. Do not say that which is untrue.

8. Do not sell the wine of delusion.

9. Do not speak against others.

10. Do not be proud of yourself and devalue others.

11. Do not be mean in giving either dharma* or wealth.

12. Do not be angry.

13. Do not defame the three treasures.**

*Dharma is the teachings of Buddhism.
**The three treasures are Truth, Immaculacy, and Harmony.

The Hindu leader Shivananda boiled it all down to "Be good; do good." Again, as overeaters, we need to eat sparingly so the body can signal to us when we are acting in alliance with those principles and when we are off course. As with most spiritual principles, these precepts prove much easier to memorize than to carry out. Our classes this week are devoted to discussions of the implementation of the precepts. We learn that small actions can change the world. As we replace the toilet paper roll when it is close to being used up, or carry out tossed cans we find on a desert hike, or wipe the lint out of the laundry's dryer, we are transformed.

Taking the vows is considered only a first step. Trying to live by them would be the "training" in Buddhism. At this first reading of the week I am caught by a particular line I'd breezed over before:

"Man stands in his own shadow and wonders why it is so dark. Yet only he can turn around."

Later, as I walk to the meditation hall, a brightly colored butterfly flies by. Is it basking in the light, but flying toward the dark? My reverie is interrupted as I pull open the heavy door to the cold, dark meditation hall.

I am on time for the first meditation session of the week. As we settle in, my mind immediately begins its rant, as I don't like sitting in the cold or in the dark.

Couldn't we meditate outside?

I think we should be more responsive to nature. As I stay externally focused, I think the nature deal is a really good argument. I want to bask in the warmth and feel the gentle breezes. I want to fly with the butterflies.

I wanna go home!

The meditation period is short and sweet. I find it amazing that after not meditating regularly for a few weeks now, I feel no physical discomfort sitting frozen in that still posture.

Well, at least I've planned my wardrobe well. Of the fifty lay trainees, four of us have fisherman knit sweaters. If I can bundle up with the sweater, I'll keep the fur-lined coat stored and hopefully avoid attention and embarrassment.

This week's schedule is much more rigorous than last time. Each day will have four hours of meditation. For one long stretch we'll be in that hall from 10:00 a.m. until noon each day.

How will I make it?

Also, there will be none of the nighttime "monk's teas" I'd so cavalierly criticized before. Instead, we'll be meditating longer. At bedtime, I fall quickly to sleep worrying about my ability to keep up.

This is a whole different ball game!

It's exciting to see so many people here.

I can get lost in such a crowd.

Most of my fellow retreatants are old-timers. They seem to know what they're doing. At the early-rise prayer service, many have all the passages and songs memorized. They don't even hold prayer books. Instead, they rattle off all the difficult Sanskrit passages as if reciting nursery rhymes in their native tongue.

During one long sing-along, the congregation offers prayers in homage to the eighty-five ancestors. This includes names from Buddha down to the present day. All congregants run through these names like they've memorized the phone book. We're not talking any lightweight names here like Luke, Mark, and John or even Abraham, Isaac, and Jacob. We're talking names like Kunagonmunibutsu, Butsudanandai, and Nāgārjuna, for starters. I am clearly in way over my head. Our sweaters might match, but we have nothing else in common.

As jobs are assigned, I inwardly gloat as my name is not on the list for *zafu* stuffing.

Had enough of that last time.

I'm sent alone, without a crew, to the sewing room to cut material for pillows.

Yay! I'm alone.

As I make my way around the cloister, I beam excitedly. *I'm sure the universe is giving me an opportunity to go inward because I won't have any fellow workers to focus on. I'll be alone with strips of cloth and my own head.*

When I reach the sewing room, my supervisor has not yet arrived to give instruction. Instead there's a pretty brunette woman ironing a monk's robe.

She quickly volunteers, "I am preparing my robes to take vows and enter the order. These are ceremonial patches I'm sewing on to indicate how junior and new I am. I will be beginning my postulancy tomorrow."

Fascinated to be in the presence of someone who, within the next twenty-four hours, will gently slip over the side and begin a journey of totally reinventing herself, I smile. "What courage."

I gaze at her neck-length bob and try to imagine her bald.

"I've been coming to the abbey for about eight years."

I want to ask her the world, but, tongue-tied, I can't seem to come up with a single question. I just stare in fascination.

She'd surely at one time been just like me, but is now crossing over. Embarrassed that she might notice my staring, I busy myself surveying the room. It's a low-ceilinged attic apartment with dormer windows, white curtains, and a sewing table, ironing board, and many white cabinets.

Before I take in much more, Reverend Muldoon shows up. She softly encourages the soon-to-be-ordained monk in her efforts with the robes. She explains the nuance of detail in how certain patches are sewn. "Put the brown one down your lapel and save blue for the shoulders. Here, make sure the crease is well ironed."

The whole atmosphere is so warm and loving and reverent.

Just then, it all comes to a crashing halt as the work supervisor enters to inform me of a job change. "You're to report to house number one to stuff *zafus*."

What?

Doesn't he see how cozy and secure we all are in this attic? I belong here. I want to stay here. We're all huddled up close and personal like Little Women *up in the attic with Beth, Jo, and Marmee.*

I stall for time. "Are you sure you don't want me to get started on this project?" I plead, trying to appear casual.

He smiles, saying nothing.

That verbal economy again.

"Do you know where house one is?" he asks without a smile.

"Sure," I mumble with pursed lips and a snotty jerk of my head. "I worked on *zafus* my last retreat"

I pout. My bottom lip starts to puff out.

Watch it. Job assignments are permanent for the whole week. Stay calm and pleasant and maybe he'll reconsider. Maybe you'll just have a few minutes up there. Maybe he'll realize this is a mistake.

I grasp at any possible straw. "Who'll cut fabric squares?"

Again, nothing back.

Dejectedly, I face the music.

As instructed, I report to house one and Reverend Joan recognizes me immediately.

"Oh, do you remember what to do?"

I'd like to punch her lights out.

No one is on vacuum yet, so I seize my chance.

"Yes, I did the vacuuming the last time I was here."

"Fine," she says, smiling. "You can get started on these."

I continue pouting until it's time for class. Since I'm totally bummed about this worst job assignment ever, I resolve to get the most I can out of the class sessions. We open with a discussion of the precepts, led by a tall senior monk with shaved head and long brown robes.

He explains, "The precepts are not to be taken as prohibitions, but as promises to ourselves. Those of you taking the vows will be making public confirmation to the world of the internal work you've already been doing. This evening, everyone will make a commitment to the precepts. There will be a more formal ceremony where each will be asked whether they would or wouldn't commit themselves to this way of life. You'll each have to declare 'yea' or 'nay.' Then we'll all snake-dance around the temple, illustrating how we must follow the Buddha's teachings wherever they lead."

Panic!

I'm not making any formal commitment. Kincaid had told me on the phone that I wouldn't have to vow to anything. I'm still Jewish, for Jehovah's sake. I can't promise to give up meat forever. I don't want to make a vow I know I won't keep.

I remember how Shreehardin emphasized that it is worse to make a commitment you don't keep than to make a lesser commitment that you will keep. I didn't even honor the tiny commitment I'd made with him. And now these would be witnessed by a multitude.

I muster up the courage to speak. "I came here to learn about the precepts, but had no intention of making a commitment at this time. What if someone yells, 'Nay'?"

Kindly, he asks, "Do you have a particular question or stumbling block you'd like to discuss?"

I can't be totally honest. I can't belt out, "I'm a carnivore."

Instead, I lie. "I'm just too new at this to even come up with a question. I'm sure I have millions, but can't even formulate them right now."

Liar!

I know that usually by the time I can formulate a question, I have the answer; however, I am drawing blanks. I certainly haven't been meditating enough to feel secure and trust what goes in or comes out of my mouth.

Well, maybe I don't really care about beef. Maybe I'm just rebelling against any restrictions of my freedom.

I'm let off the hook. He goes on to explain more about the human condition and our difficulty in keeping the precepts. "We are trying to create the least amount of harm. Buddhists believe that we naturally *want* to do right action, and have a natural tendency to let things rise and fall without attachment. Living life creates fear and, of course, greed, anger, and delusion. These all work together to develop our clinging, insistent holding on."

There's no pressure to join or take up the ranks. It's clear I haven't done any real thinking about this and don't even know enough to make any kind of clear commitment. I'm not a Buddhist. I don't even behave correctly toward my fellows. Look how I grabbed for the vacuum hose.

Tomorrow I'll offer to trade off the vacuum and take on pillow stuffing.

The evening ceremony is very impressive. Reverend Kinnett leads us in lighting candles and incense. At the introductory retreat, I had feared her ominous bulldog visage. Now, when she opens her mouth to speak, decidedly upper-crust, British, crystal tones just flow off her tongue, and I am soothed. She is calling for Buddhists to declare as she asks the whole group, "Will you keep these precepts or will you not?" I remain silent while the throng responds, "I will."

I'm busy looking down.

After this session, we're sent back to the bench for one more meditation session before sleep. My mind wanders to a distant memory I'd never recalled before:

I'm five years old. We are living in Frankfurt, Germany.

I awake, hearing a plop sound from across the wall. Plop! Plop! Splat! Crash! Shatter!

I wander out, eyes squinting in the new light. Glass shards on the floor. My parents are chasing each other around the apartment. They are both heavy people, and the walls shake when they hit.

The plops are punches.

I hear Mom's voice. "How dare you hit me, you son of a bitch!"

Then a louder crash, and all goes quiet.

After some wait, hoping someone will come to see about me, I pad in my Dr. Dentons into the dark and silent hallway. There is glass everywhere.

Dad's favorite beer stein is shattered, and its pewter lid is on the far side of the floor.

I stand in the hallway crying.

What can I do? How can I fix it? How can I make things better?

I know to head for the broom closet. I begin sweeping. The broom handle is too tall for my tiny frame, but I try to sweep up the debris. I am singing softly to myself, some kind of lullaby. I steer the shattered glass toward the red plastic dustpan.

Taking action helps me feel safe, and my crying stops. As long as there is something I can do, some effect I can have on the situation, then I won't have to cry. I can sing, even if the song is a sad one. Then things will work out.

The Beatles instructed Jude to take a sad song and make it better. Making Mom's sad song better was to be my task for the rest of her life.

And my credo became "Take action, get busy, *do something.*" Existentialists tell us, "We are what we *do,* not what we *say.*" The Christians chant, "Faith without works is dead," and the twelve-steppers tell us to "walk the walk."

But the Buddhists say, "Don't just *do* something, sit there."

Who will I be if I do nothing and just sit? Could I dare to be a human being instead of a human doing?

At the day's final meditation session, the leader is really getting on my nerves. Evening meditation is usually the most difficult since most of us are tired and somewhat distracted. There's always a lot of squirming and coughing at the last sitting. There is a special gong the monk sounds when people are getting too squirrelly. He bangs it loudly, and I assume it is to get our attention and get us back "inside." On this particular night, each time I get comfortably zoned out, he bangs on his gong.

So what if a few are squirming? Does he have to disturb all the rest of us with his obsession about those few?

I'd like to teach him a thing or two about twelve-step principles. In twelve-step circles, you hear a lot of "work your own program."

It's sort of a variation on "mind your own business," or "walk on your own side of the street."

If only he'd ask me for some timely advice.

At the end of our meditation he lets us know his irritation as he stridently announces, "Those with digital watches need to leave them outside of meditation or make sure they do not beep during sitting ceremonies." This guy sure notices every little thing.

But I'm so keenly aware of his behavior because it reminds me of mine. I have a similar external focus. Mine shows up as "theater rage." Rudeness in theaters pushes all of my buttons—especially those brats whose text messages distract me with the lit screens. Worst of all are the ladies who keep zipping and unzipping their purses. My ears prick up at the slightest whisper and I'm quick with my "sssshhhhhhs." The noisy offenders either comply or we have a fight or some variation thereon. I've threatened to bring a megaphone the next time I go to the movies, and when they start talking, announce loudly at their heads, "Please finish your conversation in the lobby." Anyway, the point is that such rude individuals are going to continue doing what they do and the meditation leader and I are going to keep plugging in and reacting, because that's what we do.

The next morning I fall asleep for the first part of the meditation session. I'm awakened by the growling stomach of the trainee next to me. My attention travels away to food. My mind concocts an elaborate recipe for a diet dessert using sugar-free pudding, nuts, and some sugar-free cranberry Jell-O. (I'll let you know how it turns out.)

Then it's time for walking meditation.

Great.

These two-hour sessions will be bearable if interspersed with some walking and stretching.

Again I get an aggravating retreatant in front of me.

This woman has no idea that there's a procession following her. She's doing fancy marching footwork, turning sharp corners, and stopping and starting out of rhythm.

Doesn't she realize the point of this is that we all work in unison like a giant caterpillar winding around the meditation hall?

Is that the point? Where did I get that? I actually made it up. But I'm sure it's how things *should* be.

I hope no one behind me thinks I'm responsible for our rotten formation.

Still enraged and externally focused, I pad back to the bench to resume sitting. Realizing how easily I become "outer" directed and reactive, I sit down to make a concerted, conscious effort to go inward.

Instead, even though it is barely 5 a.m., my whiner surfaces: *What a miserable morning this has been. Everyone was in my way in the bathhouse. Especially annoying is a young redheaded twit who brushes her hair right in front of the cubbies so no one can grab their toothpaste. She's totally unconscious. Later, as we line up to pee, she's standing in the stall blowing her nose. Without permission to talk, it seems only reasonable that I pull on her scrunchy to get her attention.*

Everyone keeps bumping into me while I'm trying to slip into yet another layer of leggings as the morning frost descends. And then the morning ceremony is led by a haughty monk I'd grown to dislike at my first retreat. Then, in prayers, the trainee next to me is showing off, reciting too fast so I can't keep up in my reading. Nothing is going my way. Everything is a struggle. No one has any consideration.

They're all out to get me!

Later, at breakfast, I still competitively race for a seat facing the window. No problem. After unfolding my assigned utensils, I notice I've been cheated out of a drying rag for after-dinner washup. I elect meekly not to mention it.

But I'm pissed. No one told me you could bring your own dinnerware and utensils. I'm stuck with a plastic child's dish with separated compartments. I also get a measly six-ounce cup.

(This cup might be appropriate for banging with the hissy fit I'm working toward.)

I could have brought that cup I got in Hong Kong with its red metal lid to keep the heat in. It has a great dragon painted on the side. Dragons represent defenders of the temple. Then everyone here at the abbey would know how smart and sharp I am.

Here I sit with resentment and regret before the first day begins. Oh, lest I forget, I'm also covetous.

All I need is a high chair to start banging my rattle.

G*reed,* **A***nger, and* **D***elusion.*

Ye **GAD***!*

She's back.

I guess I'd better take a break, slow down, and chill out. That meeting-three-assholes–in-a-day thing . . .

Tonight's ceremony will deal with contrition, and I've promised myself to deal more with amends to my mother. I keep chewing on the same bone. I know it's the meat of my meal in more ways than one. I'd spent a lot of years in therapy wallowing in self-justification and self-pity. In reciting the Serenity Prayer we ask to "change the things we can," no matter what the other guy has done or is doing.

In other words, let it begin with me.

Focusing more on what I can and can't do, and less on what those around me are doing, I get another brilliant insight. The voice gurgles up within: *"If you didn't want to get bumped around in the mornings while dressing, why did you pick the cubby by the door in the middle of the walkway? Asshole!"*

"Yeah, sure you didn't know." We all know all, all the time. Do we choose to pay attention, or remain unconscious and asleep?

Am I one of those people who set up angry, irritating situations in order to act out my rage within? Oh, please, not at this late date. I've already worked through all that.

What action can I take to stop this? I'll definitely have to offer to switch off my vacuuming with the stuffers. The guilt is killing me. It's why I'm striking out and criticizing everyone else around me.

Arriving at the workstation late, I see all my fellows stuffing. No one has grabbed *my* vacuum hose. I most magnanimously offer to switch. "Hey if any of you would like to trade off and do vacuuming, please let me know. I'll switch anytime. I know the stuffing gets tedious sometimes."

Already hidden behind masks, they each nod with bleary eyes and return to stuffing. No one takes up my offer.

It's back to basics here. Well, I've done my good deed for the day.

In the subsequent meditation, my innards begin cooking up a worry stew. Settling onto the bench brings my mind back to HOPE House and all of its problems. Has the vehicle been fixed? Did the building inspector in Hollywood sign off on the expansion? Is anyone keeping in touch with the IRS? Has the new counselor received adequate training?

I know I have to stop this mind chatter and go further in. After a few moments, I go so far in, I turn inside out. As I focus, I seem to keep on going, just like it says in the Buddhist prayers: "going, going, on and beyond."

I zone out.

My heart is pounding rapidly and my throat is dry. I'm gasping for air. In a few seconds, I can work this into a full-blown panic attack. My lips start quivering, just as they did during my first visit. Given this chance to slow down, I am shaky. As I stop all movement and thought, my lips vibrate again. Might be the cold, but I think it's the quiet.

I try to focus on my boundaries, try to feel my skin.

But there's nothing there. Finally, I find my hands, place them with thumbs touching and fingers cupped, as instructed. I press the thumbs together and they melt right into and pass through each other. All this transpires while I sit perfectly still and erect.

What's going on? My body is melting.

At the same time, some inner core of I-know-not-what keeps me sitting up straight and staring straight ahead. It has a centered direction of its own, apparently has no thoughts and no experience of any physical sensation or change. It's just there.

Who is this stone person?

I don't feel like it's me, necessarily, but it's also not not-me either. It's some being just hanging out. I know I don't want to leave this place. Besides, there's nowhere to go.

Zap. All stop.

I instantaneously feel a shock wave and see a bolt of white light in front of me. Everything gets very still. My head vibrates like my thighs would after a long race. I can feel every cell and capillary gushing blood and electrical energy. My tongue falls forward a little. I can't move even if I'd want to. I'm transfixed and solidly planted on this bench.

A wave of calm comes over me, as my body freezes in perfect stillness. Breathing normalizes.

Clarity appears on a purely nonverbal and nonintellectual level. It's a bolt of pressure into what feels like a wide-open chest cavity. I suddenly see into myself at an extraordinarily deep and grand level.

You are abusing yourself.

You are sitting in a quiet meditation hall on top of a mountain beside a volcanic crater. There's nothing to harm you and all your immediate needs are met. You are taking yourself into worry, despair, and anxiety. You have deftly transported yourself away from this safe place, thousands of miles into situations you know nothing about and certainly, at this moment, can do nothing about. You've decided to beat yourself up this morning by worrying over ongoing, never-ending, just-the-business-of-life, meaningless chatter. You are choosing to spend your morning obsessing.

Notice how your pulse is throbbing, your throat is dry, and your breathing is stilted and heavy. Your body is actually experiencing these events that may or may not be reality. While you are choosing to beat yourself up, your body is screaming, "Enough already. Ouch!"

Ouch is the only word I can muster to capture all this awareness. I start to sob.

"Ouch!" she cries again. I break into soft whimpers, with tears streaming down my face. It's all so clear. I've spent major portions of my life in this kind of self-abuse. I choose situations over which I have no control, and then work myself up into anxiety and fear.

I can do it all alone, by myself, in the privacy of my own head. Even though our business has been steadily growing, I doubt the future. We've even offered healthcare benefits to our staff and are hiring again. Does that impress me? No. I'm always after *more,* not because we have emergencies, but because I *need* emergencies.

I need to feed this pain?

I want to live in dread and fear?

I need the crises?

Obviously.

What would I do with myself should I have no crises?

This, of course, would be my personal *koan,* my life's work to ponder: could I live in a world without fear?

For the time being, I can only whimper.

It can't be true that I'm doing this—that I'm making up worry to occupy myself or make myself important or distract myself. After all, I'm official. I'm president of the corporation. Isn't it my job to worry? If I don't worry, who will? Isn't there value in worry? Why, isn't it almost measurable: equal parts worry yielding equal parts positive outcome? If no one worried, how would anything get done?

I suddenly remember reading in a management magazine about an executive who let papers lie in his "IN" basket for at least a week. Then he transferred them to an ongoing file. If no one approached him about any of them for a month, he threw that file away. He felt important things would be brought to him as needed, and most other things worked themselves out without him.

At this moment, his approach seems more than reasonable.

What does my worrying do except create anxiety and fear in others, making them less effective?

I've come from a long tradition of scaredy-cat worriers. We were taught that you actually had to measure your quota of suffering. "No pain, no gain." You could evaluate your situation like the statue of justice, using a balance scale, measuring out your investment, making sure you'd applied a certain amount of worry in order to gain an equal measure of product. Without the necessary worry stamps, you couldn't collect your prize at the end of the rainbow. You would not have *earned* it.

This brings in a whole new wave of tears. What if I am *given* a good life, not because I've earned it, but just because I *deserve* it?

But what if I give up the goo-gobs of suffering I've transited through on this journey? What about my battered childhood, alcoholic marriage, lifelong obesity, abusive parents, jealous mentors, countless chaotic love affairs? If I don't have a *story,* then who am I?

I suffer, therefore I am?

No wonder I'm so judgmental of all the ascetics depriving themselves to take on and advertise suffering. I judge every fanatic exerciser, vegetarian, celibate, or lotus-sitter. Anyone imposing pain or deprivation catches my scorn.

Why?

Because I am one!

It's difficult at first to accept this picture. After all, I enjoy such a good life, with travel, material gifts, interesting work, and two comfortable homes. But on a deeper level it's a life of suffering, because I operate daily out of fear that it will all fall apart. Since it is not a gift, I must have worked hard for it and I'd better keep on working harder or I'll lose, big time.

Where is any voice asking, "Jude, are you all right?" Truth is, I am such an important person now that I run away whenever I get near people who might ask me that.

I know if truly asked by people who really care, I'd crumble into a heap. That is what attracts me to this temple high on a hill. Here *I* get a chance to at least ask the question.

Time passes. I have no idea how long I stay like this. Then the gong sounds; time for lunch.

I end meditation in a daze. I can't focus on anything. All sights and sounds are foggy; I'm zapped into another dimension.

I get the dining hall seat facing the mountain, but I stare blankly into my plastic plate, where I slap down my food. When the bowl comes my way, I'm presented with premeasured portions of mock egg salad. I feel nauseous, thinking, "It's just too much to eat."

I don't even want to eat, but go ahead and pile salad greens anyway. Feeling passive and helpless, I want to starve right now. Any bite will take me away from this awareness. I deeply understand every anorexic I've ever treated. I feel all the violence, passion, and pain of my whole life. I want to feel it.

I eat a few bites in a fog until announcements. Reverend Kincaid instructs, "Meditation will be canceled this afternoon. You should all try to take a shower during rest period. This evening's ceremony requires our getting as clean and pure as possible.

And just when I was really looking forward to the next sitting! I want some more of that meltdown thing. It seems like as soon as I get comfortable, they snatch something away. After lunch, I welcome that coveted rest period. The mountain has clouded over, so there will be no sun in my graveyard today. I sit by the fountain to cry some more. Waves of depression invade. I'm not crying over any specifics, just seeing the whole pattern.

Self-abuse has been my whole way of life. It's what I do. It doesn't help to know more about *why*. I simply have to acknowledge that this is what I do. I manufacture chaos. In fact, my best assets surface in crisis. That's when I calm down into ninja stance, move with stealth and focus to deftly get the job done. I'm the one to have at a car wreck. I should have been a paramedic. Chaos is my meditation. It forces me to go within.

After these focused times I abuse myself with food, alcohol, overspending, chaotic relationships, or worry. But without the chaos, I'd simply cease to exist. It's all I know. Those moments are when I'm most alive.

I am finally experiencing that overriding grief and despair they'd told us about. They told us it comes when you truly take an honest look at your life. I am simply seeing the price I've paid for the life I've created. I'd like to just shave off a little bit of the worry and add on a little more compassion.

What's really being faced here is that you've abused yourself. You're a battered child with yourself as perpetrator. Sure, you can throw in some psychobabble about the "parental introject," how you learned it from parents and now carry your own judge on your own shoulder, tracing the roots back to the steppes of Russia. Who cares?

What you are facing, fully and finally, is that THIS IS YOUR LIFE.

It's not a drill, and you get no second chances.

This is *my* painful path! I have to accept it and walk it proudly and stop trying to deny it.

I don't want to face any more of this right now.

On the flight home, I can't eat or talk much. Quickly unpacking, I catch a glimpse of myself in the bedroom mirror, looking much younger. There are no bags under my eyes, and most importantly, that vertical, parallel-line crease is gone from the middle of my forehead. Instead it is flat and open with a look of the naiveté of a child. I draw closer, straining for a second look. Staring point-blank into my baby blues, directly and earnestly, I ask, "Jude, are you all right?"

She passes me a knowing, loving gaze through the tears. We both smile and bow.

Yes, I'm all right, but not for long.

FOUR
We're All One?

I'd still have to grapple with that universal oneness idea. Of all the spiritual principles, the concept of universality has always been the most difficult for me. It causes us to give up our "terminal uniqueness" and become just another egg in the carton. I failed to grasp the connection we all share. As a red-blooded Ammurrikun, I believed in individualism. I also judged others so much that it was hard to think of being a part of their group. I found my most profound lesson on this oh-so-human connection in a vomit-soaked basement in New York's Lower East Side.

For months, I'd been complaining that I had no time to develop lecture seminars and TV appearances. We had hired competent people to manage our treatment center, and were gearing up for publishing and producing videos.

I should be ecstatic.

Instead, I forget all I've learned in meditations and become excessively picky. I make no move to leave the center, getting mired down in details, demanding perfection, insisting on minor strategies to get my way. Returning from one lecture tour, I confront Robin, our program director. "Why is that fence out front down again? Doesn't anyone else care about the flower bed?" We are both well-trained professionals with people's lives entrusted to our care. My focus is on the ground. What's going on?

Because of the perspective I've found in meditation, I can't stay picky for long. I see it all too clearly with a wider lens. It looks like the last vestiges of control before truly letting go. Sometimes when you are just getting out of your own muck, something reaches up and grabs your Achilles tendon to pull you back in.

As Ram Dass said, "You've got to do it in New York." Finding a number of different temples, workshops, and sitting circles to keep myself allied with Buddhism, I like the intellectual discipline. I like the ideas. I like the quiet time. But I don't want to meditate on a regular schedule and I don't want to join any groups, and I certainly won't be regulated! I seek intermittent transcendence.

A new teacher, Jane, from Cornell, cautions, "Despite all you've done to be a Buddhist, you must meditate regularly. You must bring your herd of courageous lumbering elephants into an orderly direction. You must quiet your monkey mind to stop swinging from the vines. You must spend time settling into the eternal present of presence. Even if it's only five minutes a day, you must take time to quiet the mind. That doesn't mean chatting, writing, or even contemplating or listening to fine music. It means sitting to go blank, trying to clear the slate."

"But that all seems so glum and negative. I don't want to keep seeking 'nothingness.' I'm depressed enough already!"

Jane counters, "William James in his *Varieties of Religious Experience* had given Buddhism a bad rap, finding it a *no joy* script. That is a misrepresentation. Buddhism promotes enhancing joy by focusing on getting you most into the NOW.

"Buddha did teach about the concept of emptiness, *sunyata*. This is not about void and nothingness, but instead about the idea that things, people, feelings, do not have an inherent meaning. All things are relative and have meaning as use and interest dictate. It is true for people you know, mother, father, sister, brother. My friend is *my* friend, but to his kids he is daddy, to his parents, he is son. To his wife he's lover, provider, friend, mate, coparent. Meaning and definition rise out of utility. *We* are the meaning makers."

Jane continues, "In fact, the concept of *sunyata* is not empty, but really quite full. When you become empty of all your old ideas and ways of seeing things, you are open to filling. You must empty yourself of ideas of how things *should* look. You will feel most full, having the strongest sense of self, when you realize that all is interrelated and we are all in it together. It is not an independent existence. All life is made up of absolute relativity."

I grasp what Jane means when I think about the surface I use to hold my computer. It has no inherent "deskness" until I need it. Before then it is a slab of metal with some drawers and a fake wood top. Only when I sit down to write does it take on a desklike quality. This is also true with my success at lectures and books. All has happened not because of *me,* but because of my audience and the meanings they made. It's not about me. *They* wanted the information. *They* appreciated and applauded what I had to say. *They* were waiting at the right place at the right time, seeking the right vehicle. My job was to suit up and show up and deliver. I've been the channel and *I needed them*. I would not have enjoyed a long career delivering my message if there were not an audience hungry to hear it. My early experience at the lecture to the medical committee showed me that some magic happens between me and the audience so that we all together deliver the results.

In the late 1980s, drastic changes swept through the treatment environment. First, most treatment centers focused on anorexics and purgers and ignored overeaters. It seemed more comfortable for staff to focus on patients with more aberrant behavior, those they could hold at arm's length. If we treat "overeating," then we all have to look at our own forays into food. Second, managed care (or, as we called it, "damaged care") came to California. I found our well-trained and caring psychiatrists spending long hours on the phone arguing with insurance clerks, begging for authorizations for one more day of treatment for a very sick patient. Those same insurance companies insisted that we no longer had professional privilege, but would have to send them all client information, to be shared with employers at will. I didn't want to adapt. Those professional staffs that were willing to adjust to the new guidelines, most specifically that drugs had to be administered from day one of treatment, were able to survive. I was not totally opposed to drug help along with the megadoses of family therapy and behavior modification, but I wanted a brief first week after admission when we could get the heavily sugar-coated patients off all their excesses and see what personality was underneath the compulsive eating. I wanted to see who we were really medicating before we considered drugs.

Insurers favored drugs, which were cheaper than a hospital stay. A delicate dance ensued. Insurance companies wanted patients on drugs early so out of the hospital quickly. Our team wanted a chance to evaluate the total person. We could ward off the pill pushers for a while if the patient "refused" the drugs. We advised patients to "just say no!" This worked in some cases for brief periods. Funding was also cut for any family groups and staffings. Many centers were becoming like prisons where patients were monitored in the toilets to make sure they didn't vomit after meals. Gone were the days of encouraging personal responsibility. The medical model had won out with a vengeance. The sickness model had overshot the mark. All in all, the glory days of treatment were ending, and frankly, Scarlett, I'd been too spoiled. Our teams had been privileged to do great work, freewheeling and flying by the seat of our collective pants. It was a delicate dream, and, like all dreams must, it had come to an end.

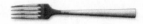

We close our doors in the 1990s and I am off to spend more time in New York developing my speaking career. I respond to a call for an interview with a prestigious agency that books big-time international speakers around the globe. Somehow hearing of my work, *they'd* called *me*!

I was wildly ecstatic, as I'd spent years auditioning for lecture agencies, finding only rejection or outfits that did less promotion and marketing than I already had in play. They charged high commissions for doing nothing. I pumped myself up with visions of "finally, professional representation."

I'll be with the big guys now: slick brochures, larger audiences, amphitheaters, the respect I DESERVE.

Soon I'll wave a hand with that wonderful, flip line, "Talk to my agent."

In other words, I'm up for it!

After a brief interview and review of my press kit and credentials, Mr. Stanton explains, "We handle mostly political speakers. We represent people who are already international names in their own right. We don't promote anyone. We just field calls for the already-famous.

"We don't really represent beginners, and self-help or healthcare have not been our strong points. We're just called for political events. We contacted you because we'd been solicited by a food-franchising firm for a speaker to help their fat employees, and this may have been a one-time project. They've since bowed out. We'd like to keep you in our files, and know we'll use you if ever we get such a request again. But for now, it's just not our area of expertise."

He gives me excellent leads on other agencies. "Please use my name as reference. I like your style and message." We part with a handshake and "Keep me updated on your new ventures so I'll be continually reminded."

All in all, a great and productive meeting. I smile all the way down the marbled hall outside his classy office, but when I enter the elevator, my face and ego sag.

I'd set myself up with such high, hopeful expectations that even though I'd gained a lot, I felt depressed. He said "NO," and that spelled rejection. Some twelve-steppers tell us that "expectations are premeditated resentments." I've found that most overeaters turn to food, not in the major crises and traumas, but over minor disappointments and expectations not met.

I am saved from overeating over this as the next day I am booked to appear on *The Maury Povich Show* and I want to have clarity and all my faculties. I'll be interviewing Marta, a dark-haired, heavy young woman who's been bingeing and vomiting and still gaining weight. Another show where I would be sabotaged by the producer.

At least Amy, the producer, did give me a slight warning—right before we went on the air! In all our pretaping discussions, we'd planned that I would confront Marta about her denial. We would have a quasi-intervention where I would try to help her see that her methods were no longer working, that she'd have to admit to being out of control and become willing to seek help.

After I've finished with hair and makeup, Amy enters my small cubicle to tell me about altered plans. "We've flown Marta's boyfriend down from Canada. In the middle of your segment, he is going to pop up out of the audience with a bouquet of roses and a ring and propose to her on the air! It's going to be so sweet and sentimental, it will be great for our ratings!"

I'm in shock.

How can we show the nation a woman who is committing slow suicide, and then joyously reward and congratulate the behavior in a media circus of premarital bliss?

A colleague later told me I should have walked out right then and there. I didn't think of it.

Instead, I thought, if you can call it thinking, *The show must go on.* And it did.

In the middle of my confronting Marta, boyfriend Ben pops up with the bouquet and runs up onstage to plant the ring and a kiss. Quickly cameras circle, audience faces are beaming, Maury is acting surprised, and my face is glum as glum can be.

What do I do now? Just sit quietly. Let it happen.

No such luck. Maury turns to me with "Judi, what do you think of this?"

The show is careening to an end with applauding audience and theme music starting up. I reply, "Maury, anyone who would choose a woman in this condition doesn't know what he is in for. Without the excess eating and vomiting, a whole different person will show up. It would be better to reconsider marriage after some kind of treatment, first getting the vomiting to stop."

And we fade to black. Roll credits. Show's over.

(I believe my comments were cut out when the show aired.)

I give my number to the new fiancé, hoping he'll call when trouble starts.

I need a meeting! The lecture agent rejection, now coupled with a terrible TV fiasco, makes me livid. I grab my directory for New

York City and find an OA meeting listed in St. Mark's Place in the Village, starting at 10:30. That's in just half an hour.

I make a hurried exit. Still made up and in full regalia, I subway across town, and then downtown. Exiting the subway, I see a young homeless man just awakening on "his" bench. I turn away and clamber up the steps to the street.

St. Mark's Place has long been a drug dealer's paradise, and though much cleaned up since its heyday, it's still full of scary action. I find the address, a whole building devoted to twelve-step meetings. I ascend the long flight of white marble steps and inquire at the desk.

"There's no OA meeting here," says the pleasant attendant.

I hand her my meeting schedule.

"Oh, that's a meeting tonight at 10:30 *p.m.*," she says. The only morning meeting we have here is Narcotics Anonymous."

"Is it an open meeting? I just need a meeting. I don't care what kind it is."

"Sure, walk through to the back and take a seat."

Well, I've never been to such a meeting. Being a "high-bottom drunk," and hanging out in beach cities or Beverly Hills and the Upper West Side of Manhattan, I rarely get to the "down and dirty" venues. This one is probably one of the dirtiest.

Folding chairs are scattered around the linoleum floor. No rows, no order, except everyone in attendance is staring toward the podium up front. All except the guys in the back of the room are hunched over their steel folding chairs, hanging heads above buckets in case they vomit again. One guy is mopping up in the back, scooting puke toward the drain in the center of the room. The floor is wet from recent mopping.

This meeting acts as an actual detox ward for those who can't get to hospital treatments. They come here to dry out cold turkey.

What in the hell am I doing here?

Will I get anything out of this meeting?

What do I have in common with these dope fiends?

The meeting is called to order and the leader announces, "Our special speaker this morning is Charley."

As he walks up to the front, I notice I'm the only woman in the room, certainly the only person in full makeup, and most likely the only one who's just come from appearing on a national television show.

As I focus back up front, I realize Charley is the same guy I've just seen waking up in the subway.

Boy, is this an interesting turn of events.

I'll take what I can. Stop judging. Sit and listen.

Charley starts by letting us know, "I live in the subway at the end of the block. No matter what, I make it to this meeting every morning. It anchors my day."

Charley sounds much more intelligent than his encrusted clothes might indicate. He's a well-spoken subway bum.

He goes on to recount some tales of his drug days. Then he tells a story that speaks to me: "I'm in this shooting gallery in the Bronx. We've just scored some good smack and are passing the needle. I'm getting quite a Jones waiting for it to get to me. The guy just before me is taking too long wrapping his arm, preparing his works. I'm getting really pissed and impatient. He finally shoots up, but then immediately keels over dead!

"The others are all stoned out. I'm lookin' at him, lookin' at the needle he's dropped, lookin' for someone to do something.

"I'm mostly thinkin', damn, if he's OD'd, I probably shouldn't try this shit.

"I'm pissed, I want my dope. I paid my share.

"In a minute I make my move.

"I say to myself, *Man, that guy always had a bad heart. This shit won't hurt me.* And so, I take my hit . . . .

"Well, I'm still here. He's dead."

Hearing this, I am just as frozen as I was when my egg cracked at the abbey. Just like then, realizing I am habituated to my own suffering, I now see that I am just like these drug addicts, just like Charley. I make the same errors in judgment every time I decide I can eat to excess. Each time I think I can binge with impunity, quickly jumping on the scale and hoping to have gotten away with something, I am doing a Charley. We're all doing it. We're all just alike.

I hear nothing else of Charley's share. I got all I needed. Right there is the essential insanity of all addiction, the pompous assertion, "My case is different. It won't happen to me. I can live recklessly and gamble and won't get burned."

Charley said it about needles and smack. I say it about cake and ice cream. We are all the same. We all use the same denial mechanisms to talk ourselves into self-destruction. We all believe we'll get away with no consequences. We all defy the laws of karma. We all gamble our lives away.

I had come from a TV studio wearing a silk suit. Charley awoke from a subway bench and walked the same block to the same meeting.

FIVE
Own the Dark

If we're all alike, I must be more like my mom than I care to admit. Now it is time to set aside my powerful public image to travel deeper within. Hadn't I been living as the "professional," hoping to escape the ghetto? Perhaps my self-image would have to find its middle path.

Mom and I have planned to meet in front of Brighton Beach's "Hello Gorgeous" beauty salon. As she walks toward me, I note she is roaming aimlessly, stopping at Korean grocers, standing in front of fruit bins, staring blankly. She approaches me with no smile and bland affect. "I'm looking to see if they have Comice pears. I like those."

Coast is clear. She's not gunning for me. I can tell the waters are safe. This would be a visit with no rage, but instead, mundane conversation.

"How's your toe, Ma?"

She's complained of a fungal infection. She smells worse than usual, that cheesy smell of fat people when mucus is caught in the folds. I remember one particularly fastidious administrator at a hospital housing my treatment unit. After following one of our extremely obese patients into the lavatory, she whispered to me later, "I think she's been vomiting."

Yes, the stall reeked of vomit, but the odor oozed from her external body, not her innards.

This visit will hold an intimate sweetness. "Let's go to the nail place and see about your toe." While Mom sits for the newly arrived Russian to minister to her feet, I go to Rite-Aid for antifungal medication. I feel no revulsion or embarrassment at how she looks or smells. Later, we go to lunch.

After some confusion in locating someplace to eat, finding only noisy, dirty places or else fancy Russian nightclubs, we finally settle on a Japanese place where I can get sushi.

"I'll order a sliced beef plate," Mom offers quietly. "I don't understand sushi."

Who really does?

She eats hunched over with her face close to the plate, using no knife, just stabbing a slice of beef, then pushing the whole thing into her mouth, first on the left side and then the right. I recall one hospital visit when she ate in similar fashion. The young candy striper came over to tell me, "Slice her meat for her."

"She likes to eat this way," I answered back.

Don't they know how people really live?

Maybe I'm the one who doesn't know how people really live.

I took my college sweetheart to Brooklyn once to meet my mother. He was from a Philadelphia Main Line family. Shortly after the visit, he found someone else. Two decades later, when we were both divorced, he contacted me, still madly in love, explaining that he had to leave me because of the sick connection he saw between me and my mother. He also couldn't take the filth.

No one could. When the social worker from Jewish Family Services called me complaining, "We've sent out three Russian maids and they all ran in horror," I didn't know what to say. She continued, ignoring my silence, "Your mother's place is filthy. What are you going to do?"

"What do you want from me?" I answered. "I have been waxing my mother's floors since age seven. I made all the meals and did all the cleaning. It doesn't matter how you clean. She wants to live this way."

But this visit is outside, so Brooklyn street smells drown out anything else. It's a bright, sunny June day, but Mom's wearing a wool knit cap tied askew under the left side of her chin. Her hair is the usual curly, thinning, straw color. She has a big smile and a slightly crazed spark in her eye.

This will be the last fun visit we have that isn't clouded with drugs and hospital staff. Little do I know this is our last chance at normalcy. So nice to have a pleasant memory.

We'll meet again at the end of summer, after I return from a lecture tour to find New York suffering through a truly record-breaking heat wave; the sexy kind, where big-hipped women stand at open windows in bias-cut charmeuse slips staring through fire escapes down to the street. There's a blackout in Washington Heights, the mostly Latino and black neighborhood housing Columbia's medical center. Electricity has been out for a week. Newscasters marvel that the residents have accepted the problems and banded together, even assisting police with traffic tie-ups.

The delay in restoring utilities forewarns the future horror of New Orleans after Katrina. Poor people rise to make the best of things, but are still serviced too slowly. Locals complain about why the international community only hears of muggings in Central Park. Cooperation and goodwill amongst New Yorkers in crisis goes unmentioned.

New York's streets are at their fetid worst on Sunday nights on the West Side when all the restaurants load black bags of slime to rot at the curb, awaiting next day's pickup. The stench assaults young couples just back from slow walks in Riverside Park, strolling arm in arm up to tiny cubbyhole apartments.

The smell of rotted garbage fills my nostrils while thoughts of personal decay plague my heart. My mother's mental illness is getting worse.

She's been hospitalized after another fall. After I've gathered needed things from her apartment, cleaning the place up a bit, clearing the floor of the mounds of old bills, receipts, bank statements, and coupons so she'll be safe not to slip and fall again, a satisfied feeling emerges.

Always better when I can find something to do.

After ordering Med-Alert, I shop to stock her fridge, lingering in aisles and at freezer cases reading labels. Trying to be the "efficient, good kid," I struggle to get all the right purchases— healthy bargains.

I really want to stay away from the hospital, feeling only helpless and irritable there, not knowing how to proceed.

I'd been contemplating my mother's death for years. As a college freshman, I'd read Camus' *The Stranger,* which opens with "Mother died today."

The protagonist goes through all the motions of making burial arrangements, always knowing he feels nothing. He's just getting through. I'd once heard a speaker describe her addicted sister's death with everyone sighing, "Thank God it's over."

Will that be what I have to say?

I would have preferred to tell the kind of good-news stories I'd seen in my family therapy groups. I'd helped so many mothers and daughters, once at odds, find a way to connect and become best friends. I wanted a reconciliation, like I'd heard from the actress Demi Moore as she described, oh-so-honestly, that although she and her addicted mother fought a lot, in the end she came home to nurse her mother and ease her way into death. Instead of such stories of joy and redemption, mine reeks of pathos and guilt.

I thought a lot about how I would handle her passing. *Would it be important to have a dramatic Hollywood deathbed scene of repentance and declarations of love? Didn't we want to have that idyllic, poignant, and (cue violins) perfectly cathartic moment? Didn't we?*

Why make it something it isn't?

When I meet with the social worker to discuss Mom's transfer to a facility for closer monitoring, he assures me she is fine. "The doctor says *irregular gait* caused the fall. We'll get her a walker, and admit her to an extended care facility for observation."

My doctor friends advise that to get a faster admission to extended care, it is better to keep her in the hospital. I try to tell her the plan, but she starts yelling and carrying on.

Afraid she'll cause them to insist on her release. I leave quietly.

Returning to Manhattan for my weekly group with the Hassidic ladies from Williamsburg brings energy back to my own life. These ladies fascinate me. Most have been referred by Dr. Abraham Twerski, a world-renowned and respected psychiatrist who has written extensively about alcoholism. They live in two worlds, half in a previous century and half in modern times, totally immersed in their spirituality. Every time I quote them some Buddhist idea, they quickly respond with "That's in the Torah." They live under tremendous pressure to get married, have many kids, and keep their weight down.

Mom calls before the group is to meet. "When are you getting out here to see me?" she hisses.

"Ma, I just got back from visiting you."

"Oh, shut up! You did not. You were never here."

I never know what is real, what is drugs, what is ranting mental illness. I admit now that I didn't know the gravity of the situation. The doctors didn't either.

I try to placate her. "I'm going into group now."

"You're always so goddamn busy with your fuckin' clients. It's time you thought a little about your own family."

"I'll be there soon, Ma."

"I'm going to die in this goddamn hospital and it is going to be on your conscience for the rest of your life!"

That is, in fact, what happens.

I wake up at two that morning, tossing with strange ruminations: *Should I go to the hospital? It's an hour away. She won't know if I'm there anyway.*

I turn over and fall back to sleep. She dies at 8:00 that morning, true to her prediction. My mother has died alone. I am now really the rotten bad seed.

For me, my mother was a great force of nature. When her breath ended, there was a great calm throughout my land. I have a strange sense of loss, and not much energy for fighting, winning, competing, proving anything. I feel gentle, relaxed, and at peace. There is no one and nowhere to fight. I know my mother loved me, despite her illness, and I know I loved her despite mine. I want to walk the planet more softly, living with my own softer side, loving her.

My mother's ill wind had filled my sails. She'd been the hurricane beneath my wings. With her gone, my already-dwindling ambition fizzles like an unknotted balloon. I'm just not interested anymore. I don't need the accolades. I don't need a crowd singing my praises. I stop plugging the media, stop booking workshops, and settle into being an everyday Upper West Side therapist. I also respond to the continuing inquiries by taking on phone clients for coaching. I dare to be average, no longer a pioneering big shot. The impetus to show off, look good, prove something, is gone.

What was all the fuss? I've often heard that silence is the only name for God.

So I become professionally silent, feeling rotten to the core, knowing I should have done more.

I have no uplifting or spiritual message to carry, no interest in teaching crowds how to identify their shortcomings, defects, character traits, or defense mechanisms. I have no desire to learn more about myself or anyone else. Though we've just released *Hot & Heavy,* I have absolutely no energy to promote the book. A spiritual look at the relationship between eating and sex? What's not to like? It doesn't sell well at all. I just want to be left alone.

SIX

Dusty Countries

I have broken a sacred commandment. I did not honor my mother. Ashamed and unsure, I withdraw further. I gradually soften enough for a very special man to enter my heart. My mother might have been happy to know him. A Jewish doctor, yet, albeit a veterinarian. Since all three of my previous great loves died before me—Peter, the college sweetheart; Howard, my alcoholic husband; and Yves, the refined European—I warn Henry that I might be a black widow.

He's game anyway.

I find a satisfying personal life and, with no ill wind beneath my sails, have no need to be out in the limelight. Henry and I are quite simpatico. I learn from him a new respect for Western medicine. He learns from me a slight acceptance of the "airy-fairy." We are both learning to dance Argentine tango! As our teacher, Miguel, instructs, "The dance is an intimate conversation between one man and one woman." We learn that it involves a careful melding of energies, a surrender along with precision, and an exquisite responsiveness coupled with paying rapt attention—while also relaxing and letting go. There is an immediate feedback loop. It's a meditation. The man takes charge. The woman must be led. She is often hanging out on one foot, quietly waiting for his next direction. It also requires a firm posture and strong abs. It combines all I've learned on my physical and spiritual fitness path.

I will invest more in one person who loves me rather than in thousands who adore me. I am reminded of a famous femme fatale's cryptic comment when asked if she'd marry again: "Why should I trade the adoration of many for the contempt of one?"

With Henry, I gain no contempt, but instead love and support, and a lot of fun. During all the years of my serial dating, choosing so many alcoholics and ne'er-do-wells, when I complained to my therapist, he'd answer, "We choose who we are." Well, I've obviously grown up a few pegs, because I choose a respectable, genteel, good-natured person.

Like me? Perhaps this phase of my life involves nurturing the *good* seed. Maybe I can give birth to my true self. I could have a personal life like all the other girls. I am no longer the nondating fat girl advising my high school chums on how to handle their love lives. This heals all my teenage angst about never having a date. Finally, I am with the attractive big man on campus—a Cornell grad, Ivy Leaguer. His attraction to me and our joy in simply hanging out erases all the childhood "fatty fatties" and all the shame of my filth-ridden past. I have no image to promote. I turn off the spotlight to live my own life.

With the luxury of semiretirement, my journey takes me to distant lands. But I have to see Ram Dass at least one more time.

The flyer announces that Ram Dass is appearing in downtown Manhattan.

I'm there!

I can't believe he still has that great laugh. In a wheelchair because of his stroke, he still looks great. We've aged together, but I don't notice mine.

He's gained weight, with a big belly like my husband, Howard, before he died.

As he begins, a guy in the back yells, "Can't hear."

"That's *your* problem!" Ram Dass shoots back.

Still sharp as a tack. His usual words start bubbling out. "We are all so steeped in the culture."

A hush forms over the crowd. We always know that in the room with Ram Dass, something profound happens. You can hear a pin drop in his presence.

He continues, "My current *sadhana* (the things I take on to meet my God, my journey) is accepting the fact that my body has turned on me. My stroke is my guru. It is teaching me to allow others to care for me."

You go, guy! Me too. Overeater. Back problems. My body has motivated me to do all this seeking. I'm not as accepting as he is.

Then, out of a clear blue sky, he starts talking as if directly to me. "When my mom died, I wasn't there. I had a deep connection with her, but I wasn't there at the last. With my dad's death, I was just performing, going through the motions. I wanted to look good. Eventually, I got tired of playing good son, so I went into playing good yogi. It was all an act."

Somehow, this sets me free. I want to run up to him and scream, "My body is turning on me too! I wasn't there for my mom either. I still do good things, though. I'm not all bad."

I want to ally myself with him.

Instead I file out quietly with the others.

When you ask a Buddhist how they're doing, a common reply is "So far, so good." They focus on the present, emphasizing process and stages on a journey. They'll rarely mention goals and end points. A *New Yorker* magazine cartoon shows two monks wrapped in blankets sitting, watching the horizon. One has just asked the other, "What's next?" His companion replies, "Nothing's next. This is it."

Can it be okay for me to just keep dancing? The tango, of all things?

Why not dance where Buddhism began?

I will go to India, consult with gurus, get some treatments for my aching back, and finalize this surrender stuff once and for all. But first, like in tango, I'll follow.

Henry is invited by the Shanta Foundation to be part of a medical team assessing the health needs of rural villagers in Burma. The country, renamed Myanmar by the military dictatorship that now rules, has just suffered another repression. In September of 2007, a peaceful protest by monks was put down with shootings, beatings, arrests, and then dispersing of the monks back to their villages. There are noticeably fewer monks on the streets of Rangoon (renamed Yangon by the same junta) than during my earlier solitary visit. Henry and I decide to get to the country early to sightsee and hang out before our trek up to the villages. Due to a change of plans, I am not able to make it to Mandalay, where I want to visit with some monk friends.

Palak, a friend of the desk clerk, is visiting from Mandalay. I show him a picture and he believes he knows one of the monks. I package up $100 in American currency and hand him the envelope, clearly filled with bills, and ask if he will try to deliver it. No one gets anything by mail. Postal services are one of the many governmental functions denied these elegant people by their repressive government. Palak gladly takes the package along with my slight tip. "Please, Palak, try your best. If you can't find him, then keep the package for yourself." I never doubt that he will do his best to deliver the goods. As much as he and his family might be suffering, he would never think to steal or lie. (Later, I return home to an email from my monk friend announcing "all cash received.")

Within a week of being surrounded with such integrity, my Western heart fills with gratitude and appreciation. These noble people make the best of things every day and don't complain and don't resent. In fact, they laugh a lot. They are no less smart or resourceful than my fellow Americans. They seem much more industrious than many of my countrymen. Still, by an accident of birth, they are offered so few opportunities to make their lives better. I am offered so much and take so much for granted.

On the three-hour ride up to the villages of northern Burma, I stare lovingly into the eyes of the Pa-O people. We're all loaded onto the flatbed of the village's new truck. The women, returning with heavily laden baskets from market, are so quietly elegant with their all-black costumes and colorful fabrics wrapping their heads. Their cheeks are painted with a claylike paste made from the bark of the Tanaka tree, supposed to prevent sunburn and considered a sign of beauty. All eyes seem to be laughing, though many cover their mouths to hide rotting teeth. Some mouths are encrusted with red dye from the betel nuts they chew constantly. This national "drug" provides a slightly euphoric effect like what we in the West get from caffeine.

The Shanta Foundation has already built three schools, has purchased the truck transporting us, and is now trying to ascertain the health situation to provide needed relief. As part of this medical mission, we are given special sleeping quarters. Again, after all these years, I'll be sleeping on the floor of a Buddhist monastery. The monks will be sleeping in the large *zendo,* each in a specially assigned space. As honored guests, we will have private rooms at each of the four corners of the upper floor. Each night we are feted by a different village chief who cooks delicious vegetarian meals served over mounds of white rice. The women and children sit easily cross-legged, staring at us while we eat. Many have never seen a white-skinned person, and most find our mannerisms quite strange. We speak so forcefully and directly, laughing and commenting a lot. The gentle villagers are more accustomed to shyness and reservation. They will eat only after the monks, and then we Westerners, are finished. Some nights we join in mutual sing-alongs. First the villagers serenade us, and then we return the favor. Henry and I offer a particularly screechy rendition of "Love Potion #9" (accompanied by Temptations-like dance moves). Since there is no electricity or running water, bedtime comes as the sun sets, and we hike up the hill to the monastery. Some villagers and novice monks accompany us with flashlights, many carting full jugs up to the water tank so we can wash up in the morning. We get the best of care. When all settle in to slumber, we are serenaded by rats screeching and racing through the bamboo floorboards of our new home.

There is no "guestmaster" here. The head monk is Punjee, who is consulted by numerous villagers throughout each day. They sit lotus as he chews on his betel nut, spitting at will, throwing the cowl of his robe around his neck, attempting to hide his goiter. His English is quite spotty, and my Burmese nonexistent. Our discussions will be confined to his asking me about my bath, "Water cold?" and my assuring him it was great while dodging his stream of red saliva. So glad I've learned from Mom to tolerate the squalid side of life. In our few weeks together, I grow to appreciate his laissez-faire attitude about running the monastery. But first I have my judgments.

I daily judge their lack of structure. Due to the language barrier, I keep it all to myself. I just want to ask, *How come monks all meditate at separate times whenever they want? Why are the younger novices playing so much kickball? Does everyone have to take a nap in the afternoon? Why aren't they assigned scripture and prayers?*

Luckily, with no communication skills, I have to find my own answers. These monks teach me that relaxation is a necessary and treasured part of life. I now have a sign in my office with the Italian phrase "Dolce fa'niente" (How sweet it is to do nothing).

One favorite afternoon pastime for many villagers is watching us Westerners at the water tank trying to bathe in cold water. We suds up our parts underneath a *longhi,* which is a two-yard swath of fabric swirled around the waist and secured under the armpits. Then, in our attempt to rinse off, a cup is dipped into the freezing tank and the water is poured down the front and back. With or without the audience, I know there are so many regions I never reached.

Why aren't they studying scripture or sitting lotus?

Ministering to the villagers turns out to be a bit more than we bargained for. It is clear from the first day, as we're greeted by hundreds of families waiting to be seen, that this "assessment" is quickly going to turn into direct "treatment."

There are desperate mothers waiting with bloated babies, trying to rouse them out of lethargy. There are many toothaches and skin rashes, and many, many backaches with accompanying shoulder pain. How can we tell these women that they mustn't carry such heavy loads in baskets suspended from straps across their foreheads? How else would they have fire to cook? And what about the five-gallon jugs of water they cart up the hills each day? They must accept the backache or have nothing to wash with or drink. *Back home in the US of A., I just go into the kitchen and flip on the gas or turn the water tap without ever giving it a thought. So blessed and unaware.*

So, we find no dengue fever, malaria, or exotic tropical maladies. These people live off the land, eat healthy fruits and vegetables, and work hard, developing strong, muscular bodies. Just like Westerners, they suffer "diseases of lifestyle." They smoke too much, don't brush or floss, and carry heavy loads. The women are most vociferous about bringing change to their villages, requesting education for their daughters, especially English classes, and no matter what, BIRTH CONTROL, BIRTH CONTROL, BIRTH CONTROL.

On our third day out into a more remote village, we are welcomed by the entire populace dressed up in finery, led by a marching band. The school children, bearing bouquets of local flowers, all wear their school uniforms of white shirts and green pants as they line up to shake the hands of every volunteer. We are overcome with gratitude at *their* gratitude as they proudly display the new cinder-block school just built with Shanta funds.

In the late afternoon, a mother and daughter present themselves for consultation. We have had excellent interpreters, but many things still get lost in translation. Suji, with dark, round eyes and a mile-wide smile, is one of the ladies who complained of back pain but also carried our firewood the previous morning. She's the one who organized a cosmetology day during which I gave manicures and painted dark-purple nails onto their work-worn hands. She is accompanied by Liel, her eighteen-year-old daughter who, according to her mother, is an embarrassment. She is quite pretty with a wide smile, long, sleek, black hair, and expressive eyes. According to her mother, she exhibits unusual behaviors. With spotty translation, we get the following story: for no apparent reason, Liel begins dancing and singing in the fields. This mother is overcome with shame and embarrassment, blaming herself while loving her daughter. For months at a time, Liel is overactive, almost possessed, and doesn't seem to care about the impression she makes on those around her. All the villagers are aghast. Then, at other times, again with no cause, the girl becomes reclusive and quiet, shunning contact with anyone.

Suji is most concerned because her own mother acted exactly
the same way, and then one day just walked away from the
village, never to be seen again. This caring mother wants to do
something, change something. I make a clumsy diagnosis. There
is so much I can't ask, as the translation is so limited. This is
probably bipolar disorder. The age of onset seems right and the
changes in behavior seem to fit. But what can I say? We have no
possibility of getting them any needed expensive medication.
Maybe Merck would pony up, donating a lifetime supply. I doubt
it. Psychotherapy is out of the question. The best that can be
done here is to try to normalize the situation.

I explain through Soe Soe, our staccato interpreter, "Many people
in the West suffer with this same problem."

The young girl begins to cry.

"We use medication to control the symptoms, and we try to
find ways to channel the upper mood swings into constructive
behaviors. Maybe we can encourage her to indulge her favorite
pastime, planting in the garden."

The mother begins to cry.

Then they look at each other and, I'm sure, stop listening to any
further translations. They are staring at each other, eyes ablaze
with tears.

And then I cry. This is my mother, myself. This is shame, hiding in
plain view. I feel so much of their embarrassment. They don't know
how to tell the father. They just wish people in the village would
stop noticing things. They want shameful behaviors to stop.

And what can I possibly say or do?

I get, in that instant, what all my life's work has been about. They
are experiencing the same shame and judgment I heaped on
my mother and on myself. It is the same pain I've shared with
every sweet overeater teen who is taunted with "I don't want her,

you can have her, she's too fat for me." It's the same judgment I suffered throughout childhood and adolescence into early adulthood. We suffer something we didn't ask for and we can't help. I can't fix it. I can't offer a magic bullet. I can't, can't, can't. I know they know more about the situation than I do. They've tried everything possible already. All I *can* do is be there, listen, give a few "me toos" and "there theres," and then push on to some behavioral tools. The best that can be done is to teach acceptance of the lifestyle changes needed for living with a lifelong, chronic, recurring problem.

I see in that moment what my message has been. Essentially, in helping families move from the "sin" model to the sickness model, I was healing shame, helping people get off their own backs. The work helped so many to "normalize" their behaviors. They realized that they were doing the best they could. They could stop feeling like such freaks in the culture, and perhaps move to feeling more deserving.

When we hear from fellow sufferers, "We know how hard it is," that strengthens resolve to do what we can. In that acceptance comes motivation to do whatever it takes to change the situation. We accept the severity of the problem, accept the monumental lifestyle and personal transformation needed, and surrender to the need to continually seek help and support. Magnifying and emphasizing *how hard it is* actually encourages us to take on the fight. Conversely, when bombarded with all the easy weight-loss solutions hawked on TV or in magazine ads, we feel we should have done this *easy* thing already. It is quite disrespectful. Instead, when difficulty is acknowledged, we promote acceptance of the struggle, respect for the difficulty, and then we can "begin at once and do our best."

In the early days of my career, I developed the professional distance to describe and comment. But things have changed. Now, I am so wide-open and feel so immediately and directly that I can hardly sit with the pain of these poor lovely people. I can't distance anymore. I can only sit and cry with them. So, it's just like I'd early learned at the abbey. As a more enlightened being, you feel more of the world's pain, not less.

And we are all a part of each other? We're in it together? I'm now truly a part of all beings—and it sucks. Limited by language and much less psychologically armored, I am not able to provide "counseling" to these lovely people. Tears are all I have to offer.

I leave the nurse to finish the consultation. For the rest of our stay with the Burmese mountain people, I stay out of the treatment rooms. Clearly, I'm not armored enough anymore. I can't counsel, can't distance, can't be objective.

Now I'm losing counseling skills, too? It's continual loss. And I don't mind. As much as I no longer relish the public forum, I can also no longer sit in quiet consultations with others' pain, either. I am completely out of the weight-loss, recovery arena. I can't continue to focus on darkness.

Others will have to face and focus on these problems. I am no longer best for the job.

But I can do yoga! My malady becomes my gift. My aching back and solutions I've found are the gifts I can share. Each evening, after our trek up the hills from one village to another, I teach groups of women and some novice monks some basic stretches. I recommend that they do less squatting and more lying down on their stomachs, stretching up into *cobra* or *grasshopper.*

SEVEN
Lean into Loving Longing

No matter what weight-loss plan is followed, there will inevitably be a longing to have more food than necessary. We have to ultimately make friends with deprivation, leaning into our longing. Leaving Burma, along with openly crying the world's tears, I still live with physical pain. Despite yoga, meditation, and even living in monasteries and doing good works, my body cries out. My breath remains shallow and I feel a gray veil hanging over my head, coloring most of my interactions. In some way I need to get off my own back, or, as I'll learn, I need to stop turning my back on myself.

I'm actually not aware that I need self-forgiving. In twelve-step programs, asking for forgiveness is reserved for Step Nine. It is advised that first we need time to take a good, honest look at ourselves. Some want to rush this process. They want to get it all out of the way, as if they'll never do anything again that needs apology. It doesn't help to admit guilt for too much too often, apologizing for taking air from the atmosphere. That is premature. Many are too eager to admit too much. One mentor noted, "You can always pick out a newcomer at a meeting, 'cause when you spill coffee on them, *they* say 'I'm sorry.'" Deciding where and when to ask forgiveness is a delicate business and usually requires guidance from a mentor. Most important is how you forgive yourself. I will find some peace only after more travels and surrenders in a Ram Dass temple in deepest India.

It happens after we travel out of Burma and through Nepal, looking for the geographic cure. We finally drop down into India, where Buddha was a prince. Born in Nepal, he traveled to India, attained his enlightenment, and then preached his first sermon at Sarnak, a short ride from Benares, the holy Ganges site where Hindu corpses are burned. I want to see it all.

When this trek first began, I told my friend Michael about leaving for India and he said, "You're going to really lose weight. I was there a month and lost twenty pounds. It's all vegetarian."

He didn't mention that he was also in his druggie days and speed and hallucinogens curbed his appetite.

Throughout the trip, I resolve to eat only half-portions at meals. *But what about that delicious roti bread with all the butter inside?* I love to watch the bakers in the streets, wrapping the dough around their hands, slamming it onto hot plates, delivering it steaming to a curbside tray.

Henry and I insist on experiencing countries from the inside out. We stay and go anywhere. No tours or guides for us. We travel light and unscheduled, roaming as our moods dictate. Thanks to our mutual flexibilities, we become citizens of the world. Most of our traveling is by overnight sleeper trains where, if lucky, we sometimes get two lower berths. If not, we climb up iron ladders to the second or third tier. We sleep with all kinds of locals, such as the Indian family traveling thousands of miles to get diabetes treatment for their aged grandma, army soldiers wrapping themselves around guns for the night, or nursing students returning to school after holiday. Most impressive, though, are the thousands on religious pilgrimages. We encounter color-coordinated swarms of people dressed alike, hanging off the sides of trains, filing into towns and marching endlessly. Many wait for days in lines, barefoot, to receive *darshan* (a blessing, received just by being in the presence of a favorite guru). Newspaper headlines blare that some wealthy devotees of Mammaji tried to cut into the line, but were quickly ordered to wait in the back like everyone else.

The noise level throughout India is ten decibels higher than in New York City. There are constant honking noises and buses, along with chanting and bells from street parades. And there is never any privacy. Whole families attend twelve-step meetings and go on doctor's visits. In movie theaters, no matter how otherwise empty it is, crowds of Indians will all congregate together in adjacent seats.

Our trek is following the Ganges as we keep heading to holy pilgrim sites. In each town we encounter men with shaved heads, indicating recent mourning. Many are here to deposit their loved one's ashes into the river. One Sikh drives his moped to the top of a bridge, stops to drop ashes out of a yellow plastic bag, then lets the bag fly as well, gets back on his scooter, and drives away. Many families jump joyously into the river. We participate in nightly ceremonies watching fires, candles, incense, and chanting.

Throughout India, at small or large shrines, *lingams* abound. These are white or black marble representations of the phallus of the god Shiva. Incense, coins, candles, and prayers are left at the statue base. There seem to be no flower-petal shrines to the female *yoni*. Women aren't even allowed to pee during the day.

Before entering each city, we consult first the backpacker's bible, *Lonely Planet,* our travel guidebook, which tells us all we need to know about guest houses, restaurants, travel agencies, sightseeing, and local customs, as well as scams to avoid. In most holy cities, like Pushkar, a favorite lakeside 1960s, Beatles hangout, a sign at the town's entrance advises travelers to "dress appropriately, do not wear shoes closer than twenty feet from the sacred lake, watch out for beggars and phony *saddhus* [holy men], avoid public displays of affection, and bring in no non-veg foods."

By circumstance, I will be forced into vegetarianism, and, while eating great plates of vegetables, will lose more weight. There's something about waiting for others to prepare it in very basic kitchens, watching everything cooked so fresh, even newly ground spices in each dish, and then eating slowly and quietly. It makes it all so satisfying. Also, I shouldn't fail to mention that everything is full of *ghee,* which is clarified butter. So, it's also a treat to slide off your chair.

In Pushkar, there are forty long marble staircases known as *ghats* descending into the sacred lake. For the next four months, I will awaken at dawn to attend morning *puja* ceremonies. Devotees come down to pray and chant and sprinkle sacred water. Some stick in a toe, some do total immersion, dunking ten times or more. After the cleansing, a man will then wash out his *doti,* wrap it back on, then slide off his undergarments *after* he's put the wet *doti* back over them to wash and put them back on as well. All wet and freezing, he'll then climb back up the stairs.

Some, like me, just say a few prayers with or without a holy man, throw in some flowers, and are done. At 6 a.m. I meet Roja, a sweet young girl who gives me the "international girlie-girl greeting." She points to my earrings, smiles, and lets out a long, cooing "niiiiiice." She sells me a banana leaf basket containing a candle and flowers for me to set adrift into the lake. While making our transaction, we both flinch at a screeching, static-filled voice blaring from a community loudspeaker delivering a sermon in English and then Hindi. Despite the scratchy recording, I make out the message: "You should not favor knowledge over devotion, neither over the other. Both are necessary and really the same thing." I'm reminded of the Charles Dickens line: "There is a wisdom of the head and a wisdom of the heart." *Isn't that truly what this entire journey is about? If I seek only heady, intellectual solutions, my body will turn on me. I'll have to think on this. But with which wisdom?*

Roja watches as I launch my flower basket into the river.

Henry will have none of this early-morning reverie, as he is back in our dodgy guest house, fast asleep. Since we make no reservations in advance, we are sometimes blessed with gigantic rooms in old colonial mansions, hot showers, mosquito nets, and delicious, included breakfasts. Other times we might endure tiny cubicles, squat toilets, breezy bathrooms, and broken windows. In the south that is bearable, but in the north, like at the "Yessir Guesthouse" in Delhi, I call down to the desk for a window repair. Two young men arrive promptly with a chair and a strip of cardboard as flimsy as a shirt box. With a bit of masking tape and much hurried, frantic instruction in Hindi, voilà, they plug our bathroom window and there's no more complaint—except Ando, the desk clerk, forgot to advise us we'd need to call down to the office to have the hot water switched on. Some nights, our showers finish awfully late.

Throughout most of India, alongside the ever-present temples, curbside devotional sites, music, incense, and praying devotees, there is a background of incessant noise and filth. It's like my childhood. All coexist equally. India is everything. You can't really describe it, because there are such contrasts. The minute you are appalled at the filth, you see someone sweeping. No matter what their circumstance, nearly everyone will offer up a large smile.

The minute you say folks are mean, someone is being kind to a beggar. It's all here. Often, though, things just don't make any sense. Why don't they finish off electrical outlets and plumbing fixtures? I'll never understand why, after installing brand-new white marble floors, some jackass spits a mouthful of that red slime from the betel nut juice, creating a gross, indelible stain. Why? Is it like our graffiti?

Anyway, is my desire for white marble floors a preference or a demand? Remember the advice from the third Chinese patriarch? So many Westerners complain of their trips to India as having too much "in your face" filth and poverty. They can't stand seeing it. I asked a policeman about how so many Indians walk away from beggars with seemingly little guilt or empathy. He said, "In our country, we look at those less fortunate and feel gratitude that it is not our lot. In your country, you look at those who have more and you live in envy."

Wandering a deserted beach near Chennai, I happen to meet Alicia, a long-limbed, dark-skinned traveler from Australia, who is in India to attend a conference titled "Misrepresentations in Ayurvedic Practice." She says, "We'll be looking at the recent proliferation of worldwide clinics opening with untrained, unknowledgeable staff."

She's the real ayurvedic McCoy. I figure she might have something of a discerning eye about these things, so I ask her, "Any ideas of some treatment here that might help my back problem?"

"You must take a yoga class from Solomon."

I'm *there.*

Solomon rides up on a motorcycle, wearing a light-blue, rather dirty warm-up suit. He's slim, about forty-five. He leads me and Kao, a Japanese girl, to the roof of the Shoreline Hotel. After some initial breathing postures, he moves to helping us individually contort into pretzels. He moves my limbs and I yell, "*Nay mumkin!*" (impossible).

He says, "*Mumkin,*" and proceeds.

I can't tell you how or why, but afterward my body is light and airy. He does some shaking of the legs and stretches, similar to Thai massage. He pushes me past my edge. You know the skinny models who double-wrap their crossed legs? Well, somehow, he takes my short thunder thighs and wraps my legs like that. "*Nay mumkin!*"

At one point, as I groan in pain, he says, "I don't listen if you *beep* [cry]. I must fix! You can *beep*. I won't care."

What a pro!

He's pushing me past my limit. Just like at the abbey.

I tell him about all I've been through with Western medicine and how only physical therapy and yoga seem to help.

He responds, "Allopathic medicine only solves short-term problems, but doesn't cure. Yoga fixes you for life!"

And I've been fixed! Midway through the session, my breathing is much more relaxed and blood courses through my veins. Relief is imminent. My pain is subsiding.

As he shows me new ways to get my breath in order, I wonder why he himself has a slight throat irritation. That voice gently puts me in a trance with "IINNNNNNNHELLLLLL . . . (long pause) . . . EKKKKKKKKTAAAAALE."

He's definitely from Shreehardin's long-exhale tradition, emphasizing proper breathing more than posing. "Stretch the shullldddderrrrrrr. . . . Lock the feeeennnngrrrrrrrrrr . . ."

After our customary "*namaste*" to end the session, I ask Solomon if he has any special advice for me for the back problem.

"Just keep practicing," he advises.

"As we get older," he continues, "things just stiffen up. Even though yoga is the best for the aging process, we still age."

I really don't like what I'm hearing.

He continues, "I used to be better at the back bend, but have lost some flexibility."

"I'm surprised," I answer. "I thought when you practice more, you get better, more limber."

"Yes," he replies, "but you still age. I was a champion, but then I focused on leg work and lost what I was able to do with my back. Little children can twist into anything, but as we age, we stiffen."

"I guess it's a full-time job," I reply with a bit of a pout forming. Really, for him, I guess it is a full-time job.

And he still struggles and can't contort as he once could?

Is it continually more work with fewer results?

I remember a scene early in my weight-loss journey of watching a television host interview a still-pretty former Olympic ice skating champion. At that time her Olympic career was over, but she starred in a top commercial ice show—and she *still* practiced five hours each day to perfect her act for the weekend performance. On Friday nights, everyone, including the star, was required to weigh in. "Sometimes I just didn't make the weight," she told the incredulous host.

I couldn't believe it either. *Skating twenty-five hours a week and* still *not thin enough?*

Then I thought, *If she has to work at it, why shouldn't I?*

It was an important moment. I stopped looking for life to be fair.

Just do it!

Before leaving, I ask Solomon, "Can you advise me where to get a massage to help loosen this painful backache?"

"You might get help from Balaan. He is ayurvedic doctor. I will call him for you."

Within a few minutes, I am set for my 7 p.m. appointment.

Dressing for my massage, I decide to go braless in the spaghetti-strapped linen dress just purchased from a street vendor. I wear panties underneath, hoping that's all I'll have to drag onto an expected dirt floor.

But Balaan's floor is not dirt. His studio is on the second floor, above the Sunrise restaurant, opposite the beach temple I'd sat in all day.

Balaan welcomes me into his treatment room. He is a small, very thin and dark, attractive, mustachioed man of thirty. "I have been administering this ancient ayurvedic medicine for twelve years, and naturopathic for the last three," he says, beaming proudly. "I will take my exams next year. Last year's tsunami and our recent floods have set back my business for a while."

He is talkative and exuberantly eager to explain his work. "I waken at 6 a.m. to pick necessary herbs and plants from the forest outside of town, and I begin treatments with my first client at 7 a.m., then I am booked solid until 10 at night.

"You are lucky I could fit you in. It is only because you are a student of Solomon."

I'm feeling a bit guilty, because actually I've just had the one lesson with Solomon. I don't really qualify as "student." However, I let it pass.

Balaan is not dressed in long robes and beads, has no yellow and red dots on his forehead like the phony-baloney guy down the street. That guy blocks the footpath, setting himself up like a one-man gauntlet, hawking, bowing *gassho* continuously, sweetly inviting passersby into his incense-laden lair. I had stopped there on my way, seeking the *steam bath* promised on his sign.

"So sorry, missus. Tsunami broke our pipes and no money for fix."

Balaan instead wears neatly pressed, light-gray slacks and a "wife beater" T-shirt. He's covered from chin to floor by a green rubber grocer's apron.

He leads me in under his roof of thatched sugarcane leaves, all geometrically placed and interwoven to keep the inside dry. The small room is dominated by a large massage table covered with a flower-patterned plastic oilcloth. It's just like Mom's. At the far end of the table is a folded dirty towel for my head.

The table is illuminated by India's customary long, fluorescent light bulb with no cover. Dangling four feet down from the fixture and stopping just above the table is a large, many-legged spider.

Sure that Balaan will be swatting away the arachnid before beginning my treatment, I ask, "Do I take everything off?" I'm a little nonplussed as I see there is no cover sheet on the oilcloth. There is also no candlelight, chanting, or incense, just the natural sounds of the sea crashing gently close by.

Balaan gestures for me to undress. "Okay to leave pants if small."

Not knowing what that means, I quickly pull off the dress to reveal my lavender tap pants, which are slightly hip-hugger—not quite reaching the waist, but covering most of my bum.

Balaan waves his hand. "Take off, too big."

I quickly comply, and in a flash am stark naked, faceup on the table, staring at that hanging spider. Expecting it to fall any second, I point it out to Balaan, who answers, "Yes, nice spider, living well." He makes no move to change a thing.

Overcome with embarrassment at lying there so exposed, I become quite medical, explaining my back and leg pain and how the MRI shows severe arthritic compromise at the levels of lumbar five and seven.

"Yes, yes, I will look," he responds, ignoring me completely as he turns to the nearby gas burner, draws from a large box of safety matches, and lights the flame. He is heating oil and herbs. I decide to close my eyes and RELAX!

They immediately spring open as a small dot of oil is placed first on my forehead, then on each of my nipples, at the top of my pubic bone, on the palms of each hand, and then on the soles of my feet.

"Oops," I'm screaming inside, though my outward appearance is deeply meditative, with a fake smile of contentment.

I think I'm in over my head.

I close my eyes to blissfully dream and hope for the cure. Balaan explains, "You have what Western medicine calls a chronic, progressive problem. Western doctors will give up or cut, but it can be totally cured by ayurvedic treatments of twenty-one days done three years in a row. Before I begin on you, I suggest you come back for the next two years."

Is this guy nuts?

"I know you must leave on journey, so will just give light massage and hope for best."

I try to relax. Say nothing.

The massage actually progresses quite well. Gobs of warm oil are spread everywhere, and as embarrassment wanes, I begin to enjoy the rubbing and smoothing. I figure if I keep my eyes shut, no one will see me.

Balaan explains, "I will do only moderate pressure, as you leave tomorrow. If I do too much, all the pain will come to the outside and we will have no chance to treat it further. If you stay for full treatment, I would proceed differently with stronger pressure."

I am grateful for the moderate pressure. He begins a rotating, kneading motion on both of my breasts. Whenever he travels out to the perimeters, he seems to return to these relay stations. His hands travel up, down, and around my stomach, legs, and arms, and then back to the rounded orbs.

There seems to be more than one set of hands on my body. The man has miracle fingers. At one point I wonder, *has someone else entered the room?* When returning to his hot oil pot and bottles, he maintains one hand on my body at all times.

He spreads these potions across my back and down my legs.

Later on, reading the brochure (I'm always one for jumping in first and reading directions later), I find that a deeper treatment, the three-week experience, might have included "fasting, enemas, colonics," along with oil up the nose, in the ears, and dribbled on the forehead. According to the brochure, these treatments promise alternate cures for "diabetes, heartburn, mental disorders, obesity, headaches, joint and gastric problems," and countless other ills.

At the end of my massage/treatment, Balaan produces a pouch made from a rag wrapped around leaves and herbs. He heats it, and then pounds on my back in an ordered, rhythmical progression up and down my spine.

It is soothing, and feels truly like some "treatment" might be happening. I later buy a bagful of his crushed herb powder.

While receiving these ministrations, I decide to do a little research. I ask Balaan about ayurvedic treatment for obesity. As you may know, its naturalist philosophy is a lot about balance of body, mind, and spirit. His obesity treatment is quite straightforward: "We cleanse your body of wrong toxins, and then recommend eating correctly and exercising, especially yoga."

Now there's a novel idea. *Diet and exercise?* Nothing new under this Bengali sun.

I leave Balaan refreshed and lightheaded, but the next day my back feels worse and my sinus headache and slight throat cough have returned. So much for the moderate pressure.

I try Vicodin two nights in a row, with absolutely no effect. The pain won't quit, and I need to sleep!

EIGHT

Honor Your Incarnation

I'll try purification in Puri. I first learned about the ancient holy city of Puri in the 1960s from Ram Dass at a theater somewhere near the Hollywood sign. He spoke of receiving major *darshan* in Puri. But in those days he was still allied with his buddy Timothy Leary, and they may have both appreciated Puri as a city where *gonja* smoking is still legal and served on restaurant menus in a *lassi* (yogurt smoothie). The marijuana plant is smoked in some religious ceremonies at Puri's Jagannath Temple, one of the holiest in the world. Westerners are not even allowed to enter. I found a window on the highest floor of the library across the street where you can look down into the temple and watch the *doti*'ed monks lighting incense and taking offerings.

I'd been warned—but didn't listen—that my back problem would be chronic and intermittent and might return despite yoga and my best efforts. It returns in Puri with a vengeance. I am not able to walk around the temple, as my pain is excruciating. Now I can only take three or four steps before needing to sit. I usually find a cart in the road next to the cow dung plops. Sometimes I beg a merchant to let me use his stool for a few minutes until I can walk again. I am grateful when Henry positions me on the back of a motorcycle and we make it through most cities just like the locals.

I never find a comfortable standing or lying position. I am unable to walk, not realizing that my body is signaling my soul's cry for relief.

Our hotel is a three-story guest house full of European and Australian travelers, some of whom have been there for months. Hans, a colorful neighbor, is a very roly-poly German whose wife wears eight inches of silver bangles up her arms. Hans tells me, "You need to see Dr. Dash. He's the best. His clinic is in the center of town." Miranda, exotic, tall, lean, and dark-haired, nods in assent, causing her assemblage of silver wrist baubles to clang melodiously.

I sit on a large rock outside the hotel until a rickshaw driver happens by. I say, "Dr. Dash," and he immediately smiles. "He number one. Clinic professional . . . woman with woman." I'd heard some strange stories from other tourists.

Dr. Dash is sole owner of the Ayudwar Clinic. Its brochure promises complete cure from diabetes, stroke, mental illness, and skin ailments through methods such as enemas, therapeutic vomiting, and some massage and herb treatments. I opt for anything noninvasive.

Dr. Dash is short and round with a medium-gray shirt, khaki pants, and a large handlebar mustache matching his jet-black hair. His office is adorned with pictures of Sri Aurobindo and his French protégé and lifelong companion known to all as "Mother." There are also posters with quotes from Yogananda. I smile in recognition, pointing to the pictures and bowing *gassho*.

"You are a devotee?" he asks excitedly.

I sheepishly reply, "Well, somewhat. I have been following Ram Dass since college in the sixties."

"We have an ashram right here in Puri that Ram Dass founded," he says excitedly.

Before I can go on, what with all our mutual broken English, somehow Dr. Dash gets the idea that I am a friend of Ram Dass. I try to explain, "I've been a devotee and follower. I attended retreats with him in Los Angeles, Mt. Baldy, and even New York. In Palm Springs, as a radio personality, I did a phoner with him once. But he's really not a friend per se."

Dr. Dash directs me up onto his exam table with "I'd like to talk with you later, but now, let's begin your treatments." He pokes me hard in the bowels and chest, and has me raise straight legs slowly until I find the level of back pain. Then he asks many questions about digestion and elimination.

At last he prescribes a regimen of two weeks of "juice fasts, irrigating, and enemas."

"Oops!" I gasp under my breath. "I can only commit for two days of treatments, as I'm leaving for Benares."

"Oh, ayurveda is a lifestyle change. It can't be rushed. If you only have two days, I will recommend vigorous massages with herbal poundings, and hot wax treatment."

I'm still game for anything to relieve the pain. Maybe his massage will be the breakthrough.

I'm led into a grimy treatment room by Hosha, who, oddly enough, has the first case of body odor I've sniffed in all of India. She's a tiny, attractive woman sporting large, round, Gypsy-like golden earrings. She first gives me a sitting-up massage, pounding and pulling into the core of my being. She applies pressure to different areas of my feet, upper and lower, and manipulates my joints, causing my tailbone to vibrate. Most of her focus is on kneading down that outer calf where my major ache lives. I guess she knows her stuff.

This massage room has no spa finery. The waiting room is lit by yet another uncovered fluorescent light bulb. It shines down onto dirty walls sloppily painted in high-gloss sheen. The lower three feet of wall are painted a stripe of dark blue. The next four feet up are covered with a medium shade of the same color, and then, toward the ceiling, we see a foot of light-blue paint. I guess we're going in stripes from the sea up to heaven.

The treatment room has the same striping pattern, but in dark-to-light yellow. The cabinets are stained with black finger marks and grease. I soon learn why, viewing a pot of hot oil bubbling on a gas Bunsen burner beside the bed. This creates great rings of smoke, and the room has no ventilation. Hosha has placed me on the "bed," a rubber mattress atop a large table. She rubs, pokes, and jabs as she kneads all my flesh. She's careful to stay clear of the breast area except for two quick swoops across on the way to my sore shoulders. It's that left rump, thigh, and leg that she has to press with all her might. I wince and whine throughout, though believing it is all worthwhile. She pounds and rubs with a heated, herb-wrapped hammer just like Balaan's.

After the oily massage, I'm left on my stomach. Hosha leaves the room and returns shortly with two bottles of oily red liquids and a two-inch-high ring of what looks like cookie dough formed into a large, doughnutlike circle.

"It looks like the dough that's pounded to make *chappatis*," I say, laughing. "Are you going to cook bread on my back?"

She grunts.

I do, in fact, turn out to be the griddle. The dough is placed in a circle around my sacroiliac, and Hosha kneads the ends into alternating circulating crimps resembling outer pie crusts. With this pie dough ring now created above my sacrum, she pours the oils onto my flesh and wheels a heat lamp over to shine down onto my derriere. It quickly heats up while my outer leg begins its vibrations again.

I'm hurting and want to change position. Hosha places her hand firmly on my shoulder and says, "You sleep!"

But I have to contort to change the angle of my leg, seeking some relief. I want so much to be a good patient while also trying to keep the oil from oozing into any waiting crevices.

She calls in Dr. Dash, explaining to him that I am still in pain and won't stop moving. He surveys my bare, oily bottom and whispers over my shoulder that he'll be giving me some pain pills in addition to the natural ayurvedic potions he's already prescribed. I grunt painfully as he leaves.

Hosha, trying to divert my attention and stop my moaning, tells me of her cheerful outcome. "Dr. Dash cured my back problems, but I had the twenty-one days of enemas."

No thanks. Plumbing at the guest house isn't number one, and not so easy for number two, either.

After two hours of manipulation, but before any ingestion of the prescribed potions and relievers, my pains are slightly less. I am nowhere near well by any means. Dr. Dash invites me back to his office.

"Now, we must talk some more," he begins, as those piercing eyes of the Mother poster look down intently.

Dr. Dash asks, totally out of the blue, "Have you experienced any loss?"

I begin to cry softly, gulping back a bit. "My mother died, then my stepmom, and my father died a few months ago."

"Some of your pain is happening now because it is psychosomatic. Yes, you are traveling and lifting your baggage and sleeping on trains, but you are also mourning. Your back aches for you.

"You are in an acute stage now, so we can only treat you very minimally. You need mostly rest and quiet, and you must also lose more weight."

This is said offhandedly, like it should be an easy project.

"You have no idea, Dr. Dash, how much that is an issue in my life. I live with this issue twenty-four-seven, and it's even what I do for a living."

He probes further about my work, my writing, my beliefs. "You have been published?" he asks joyously. "I have clinics in Switzerland, Rome, and a new one forming in Germany. Perhaps we can somehow work or write together to bring ayurvedic to the West. Maybe you can help me get my work more known."

He thinks I'm a publisher?

I promise I'll help all I can, but an uneasy misunderstanding is brewing.

"Many in the West want to know of our treatments here. I have met Ram Dass twice when he was here to visit. One time I treated his hand, and also looked at a sty in the eye of his assistant, Mirabai. He funded a new temple being built right here on the beach. Tomorrow I will show it to you and take you to lunch at his ashram."

Before I can protest, Dr. Dash is on the phone making arrangements.

Then he comes back to me. "I believe I have done for you all I can in this short period of time. I will give you some homeopathic tablets, but am afraid you will hurt for a while. For one thing, you must make some resolution about these deaths.

"Most importantly, you must cry. You must tell me about the deaths."

I feel awfully tense. *What does he want to know?*

"Well, my stepmom was an elegant lady who worked for the US Foreign Service in outposts throughout India and Greece. Dad married her 'cause he said she really cleaned up his act. She made him want to be a better man. She showed me how a woman could have a life without children, have fun, and take care of herself. She wrote the book *Backstage in the Great War,* about her escapades in London during the bombings and then after World War II. She was elegant, a bit aloof, and lived to age ninety-seven. Less than a year later, my dad followed her in death. He'd been a man who really, really loved me, encouraged me to be strong and independent, valued and nurtured my intellect. He so believed in our country and its values that he'd written advisory letters to every president who'd served during his lifetime. He was one of those brave men Tom Brokaw named "The Greatest Generation," a proud American and a loving father. It was a great loss to watch him fade."

"And what about your mother?"

"What about my mother?'

"Hasn't she passed away also?"

"Yes."

. . . . . .

"And?"

. . . . . .

I don't want to talk about it.

. . . . . .

Dr. Dash doesn't stop. "If you want to face your back problem, if you want to lose your weight, you must seek different answers from the ones you've had. I'm sure you have heard of the quote that a problem can't be solved by the same mind that created it. New thinking is needed."

I decide to blurt it all out. I tell many gruesome tales. Then, the worst of it.

"I wasn't there when she passed. I stayed away. I felt cold and scared."

My crying begins as Dr. Dash pauses and then speaks.

"You weren't physically in the room with her, but you were probably more *with her* throughout both your lives than anyone ever has been. You appear to be such a *present* person that I can't imagine you weren't there."

"But I don't think that counts for anything."

"Counts? Who's counting?"

He waits while I don't answer and then says, "Do you know Ram Dass was not physically present when his mother died?"

I answer, "I knew he was very connected to her, as even though he was in India when she was diagnosed. His guru heard the word *spleen*."

Dr. Dash continues, "He wasn't there at her death because he was with Timothy Leary at a psychedelic conference in San Francisco. He was living his own life."

"Yeah, but I was just in bed, sleeping. And besides, I had hatred and meanness toward her. I wish I didn't, but I did. What about *ahimsa?* (*Ahimsa* is the doctrine of nonviolence brought to the world stage by Gandhi and then practiced by Martin Luther King during the American civil rights movement.) Even though I'm trying to be a better person, where was my compassion for my own mother?"

Dr. Dash finally gets a word in. "*Ahimsa* does not mean don't fight or be stupid. One must defend. Your mother was ill. She was rageful and attacking. You found your best ways to protect yourself."

"Yes, but I am a therapist. I should have understood. I know I couldn't have saved her, but I might have helped her to feel better. I could have been kind."

"Yes, your life's work has been about helping others to feel better. You are giving kindness to strangers."

Just like Mom always said.

"Yes."

"And death is death. We each must face and do it alone. It is *life* that we can share, *life* that we can celebrate and enjoy together.

"You and your mother were locked in a kind of fairy-tale myth. Mom played out the wicked witch so that you could be the fair maiden."

"Well, I wouldn't go that far. I'm not such a sweetheart. Look what I've done. I violated a sacred commandment. I did not honor my parent."

"I think you spent much of your life trying to honor your mother, but the person who showed up as your mother was stricken with painful mental illness. That was not your soulful mother. That was a poor, sick, and suffering being who really wanted to love you. She didn't mean to hurt you and she surely didn't want to behave the way she did. She couldn't help it."

He looks down at our locked hands and then up at me again. "You couldn't help it, either."

What? I'm an existential therapist! We take responsibility for our actions.

I respond, "There was no real provocation for me to be so cold. She wasn't really on the attack at the end. I was just on the retreat. I had become mean."

"Judi, neither one of you was mean. You were both stricken with forms of illness."

And hadn't so many shrinks tried to convince me that my mother was ill? Yes, she was supposed to be the mother, to protect and care for me. I was angry that it was turned around. It was such psychobabble, blah, blah, blah. Had I ever accepted her mental illness on a deep and psychic level? It was all normal for me. It was our life together. It didn't matter what all the therapists and friends told me about how sick she was, how I did my best. Had I ever accepted it in the tissues of my being? Had I accepted it in my aching back? Had I ever deeply accepted that I was also ill? With all my great intellect, I was just coping and giving lip service, not really leaning into the pain of how sad our song really was.

"How could it be that I, someone so pretending to pursue the spiritual life, so responsible, so 'caring,' could not see my own mother's disease? She wasn't just addicted, but actually suffered delusional mental illness. Why didn't I try to talk with her doctors? Why didn't I find out more about the drugs they'd prescribed? Why?"

I drop into more painful sobbing, but don't stop rattling on. "She was so right. I helped thousands to be compassionate with themselves. But for her, all I offered was judgment and battle. I didn't know how to make it right. I didn't know how to help."

My tears flow freely, with large gulps for air. I can't breathe some of the time.

Dr. Dash lets me cry a while and then offers, "You couldn't really let it in until the siege had ended. You couldn't hold the tremendous closeness you had with each other, the love and caring, and also the horrific tragedy of mental illness. It's just too much to bear. You were too vulnerable. It would have taken a superhuman healthy ego to have the perspective to see the whole picture, the love and the tragedy. You tried, but you were only a human being."

"But I'm a therapist," I offer back, as if that should render me more powerful, but then also more guilty.

I drop into my own ruminations: *If I accept that she was truly ill, then maybe she really didn't want to treat me the way she did.*

Dr. Dash continues, "What if neither you nor your mother could help it? Aren't you also a family therapist teaching others the *systems approach*? This was your system. You were perfectly balanced in this tragedy. Your mother's life was a run-on sentence of psychosis. Yours was a constant struggle to stabilize yourself and try to distance yourself from it. You became a helper trying to understand it. You were so afraid of entering her world that you hardened your heart. You couldn't help how you behaved, either. You have to give up all your judgments of how anyone *should* have behaved. You were both in a trance."

"You mean we were both *powerless*?"

He offers no answer. Verbal economy again.

The word hangs like a suffocating cloud engulfing the room.

I stop crying briefly, thinking, *What would my "do no harm" Buddhist friends have to say about this? I am so, so disappointed in myself and my efforts. How could I have any message of hope and progress for patients when I see where all the training, good therapy, and spiritual questing has brought me?*

Those judgments ease a bit as I breathe in and feel bigger, though softer, than I ever have in my life. My body floats and expands as if I am a rubber vase filled with new, clean water. I feel expansive, large enough to hold the bigger picture, the painful reality of both love and hate and powerlessness. I think of two powerful women I've admired for years, Gloria Steinem and Marilyn Monroe, both with mentally ill mothers. Did they face any of my feelings right now?

After the Los Angeles earthquake, a friend whose house had been totally demolished shared with me, "I always knew how strong I was, but I never knew how weak I was." That's what I am feeling now. The journey has brought me down to bedrock, to weakness, not strength.

Before we close, Dr. Dash offers a homework assignment. "Before you sleep, it would be wise to take some time alone to think about your mother and all the great gifts she has given you. When you live in gratitude about how you have benefited, then you can have compassion for both your mother and yourself. Then you will feel true *ahimsa*."

I know I will first have to acknowledge the ways I am like her and see what I've gained from our struggle. I'll have to face that despite my efforts to appear different, I am, in truth, quite a bit like my mother. I'm adaptable, a great bargain shopper, and have a lot of fun with a lively wit. I've channeled through her all that exquisite Jewish humor like my favorite, George Burns, or Mel Brooks, Neil Simon, Larry David, Jerry Seinfeld, Don Rickles, Mort Sahl, Richard Wright, Joan Rivers.

I'm also a fierce fighter! Just like Mom. What I'd label in her as "stubbornness" I'd accept in myself as "tenacity." Agreeing to call mine "stubbornness" opens up deeper compartments. I'm in a submarine coming up from a dive, opening up each cell of the ship. I have to open it all up to soar out of the gutter. I'll eventually have to agree with the old folk saying, "There is so much good in the worst of us, and so much bad in the best of us, that it ill behooves any of us to find fault with the rest of us."

The next day Dr. Dash arrives at my hotel and whisks me onto the back of his motorcycle to head for the ashram. We are greeted at a back-alley courtyard by three orange-clad monks in skirts and with yellow-painted foreheads. They are naked to the waist.

As Dr. Dash had been delayed while consulting on a diabetes case at his teaching hospital, we are late to lunch. Monks are already seated on the ground, eating. He takes me to the garden hose to wash up and then shows me where to sit while waiting for the monks to finish.

The place is in no way inspiring or serene. A cacophony of cawing crows, beeping rickshaws, honking cars, cowbells, bike bells, and shouting vendors wafts in from the street. A few plants live in clay pots situated nicely in the well-swept earthen courtyard. The yellow-gold walls are worn and dirty and the decor is standard concrete block throughout.

I am dressed up in my new skirt, specially made blouse, and slippers easily shucked for entering temples. I am trying a new underwear experiment, which upon learning we'll be sitting on the ground suddenly seems like a very bad idea. I haven't even mentioned the details of latrine practice in this part of the world. If you've traveled to the third world, you know that latrines are mostly holes in the floor, with "modern" ones sporting porcelain, usually wet platforms for you to anchor your feet on while straddling the hole. Ladies pull up their saris, settling naked bums over the dirt or porcelain. They don't have to bother with underwear. Afterwards, there will usually be a small cup in a pail of water or a continually running faucet for rinsing with the left hand and then air drying. Sometimes you'll find what an expatriate schoolteacher friend referred to as the "ass wipe hose."

I have decided on this day to wear my new long skirt sans underwear, so that if the occasion arises, I can air dry like the rest of 'em. You see, in most facilities, if you try for Western practice, you are plagued by what to do with the paper and the underwear, and how to keep pulled-down jeans from settling onto the wet floor.

So, I am now joining the monks, sitting on the ground with nothing underneath my skirt. Crumpling my weak hip under me, ever fearful of which way my legs might splay, I make it down with dignity and modesty intact. I am grateful as Dr. Dash explains and apologizes for my failure to sit lotus, as I'm keeping one or both legs extended to avoid more pain.

Banana leaves are spread on the ground for our plates, and large mounds of white rice are doled out, then covered with dal sauce, vegetable fritters, and one stir-fry of green beans and another of cauliflower. No utensils in sight, I follow my doctor, cupping all in the fingers of my right hand. As we eat, a procession of monks keeps filing by to smile warmly, bow *gassho,* and stare a bit. Dessert is a delicious runny rice pudding.

After lunch, six resident monks surround us, listening in, catching whatever parts of English they can grasp. They stare and smile at me often. I guess Dr. Dash has explained that I am a "friend of Ram Dass" as he passed around my postcard showing my books and credentials. I'm treated like royalty.

We speak of our mutual treatments for patients with obesity and diabetes. Aside from the "eat less, exercise more" prescription we'd all been reciting like mantras of the modern age, Dr. Dash offers an idea rarely mentioned in Western medicine.

"It's about timing. You must consider the time, the season, the state of affairs, the state of your body. For example, *now,* because you are in acute state, I tell 'no yogurt, no cold, no fish,' because that aggravates your pain. That does not mean for all time. When pain is gone, yes, you can have yogurt, you can eat cold."

Wasn't I fighting for more flexible treatment plans? Couldn't food tolerances change with different life circumstances? Can't Western medicine consider issues of timing more?

"Also, in the West you expect quick recovery and immediate response to medication. We offer treatments of one week to three weeks, just to cleanse the toxins out of your body. For lifelong cure, it takes years to change the lifestyle. We don't expect such immediate results."

Dr. Dash continues with complete assurance about everything he has to say. "We must unite technology and history. You in the West have great tools for diagnostics, but know little about treatment. We in ayurvedic know treatment, we *have* the remedies. We can *cure* any problem."

My Western, "show-me-the-double-blind-studies" mind winces when he so cavalierly mentions "cure."

But let's face it, I'm the one with the aching back, and I do know that my physical pain has something to do with emotions.

Soon, it's time for us to walk to an upper room of the ashram to see where Ram Dass's guru lived. He had just died at 102 years of age. I truly expect a lavish shrine of some kind as we ascend the concrete steps. We're led down a modest veranda past more hand-stained and weather-beaten walls to a bedroom housing a small dresser and a hospital bed covered with an orange spread pushed against the wall. Situated across the bed are three large, three-foot-by-four-foot color photos of some older men. The pictures are draped with orange cloth along the bottom half, just allowing the faces to peer out. When we enter the room, Dr. Dash drops to his knees and touches his forehead to the floor. I do the same, a little fearful about the rear view. When we return to standing, Dr. Dash explains the lineage of each man and whose guru was whose, going back about four generations. The room has been left as it was when inhabited, and is a highly honored spot. Monks are standing outside the door, watching and smiling.

In facing the squalor, lack of decorative art, and simple "thereness" of these surroundings, I am transported to my roots, the tenements where I'd spent much of my childhood. In Scranton, the coal-mining capital of Pennsylvania, I came back courtyard. The Cannery Row atmosphere of the buildings housed such life, from the drunken bleatings of couples leaving Chappie's Bar to the Irish lady always trying to sell her chubby, carrot-topped little two-year-old girl, to the teenage bobby-soxers kissing in the underpasses between the buildings.

This ashram feels like that. In fact, all of India feels just like that: dirty, teeming with life, not decorated, and no one noticing. Life is fully in-your-face, with little facade. Accept it. Be it. Love it.

I thought of Ram Dass, essentially a nice Jewish boy with a great comic sense, though his New England background is much richer than mine. He made a break from his past. As he sought his own growth, returning from India draped in his toga and sandals, he commanded little respect from his own family. His father called him "Rum Dum" and his brother called him "Rammed Ass." I imagined him just sitting in that courtyard and watching, taking it in.

And I can take it in, too. I suddenly love my life, love my history and background. I truly love my poor, psychotic, sloppy mother and how hard she tried to keep it together. She helped me adapt to squalor. As I've traveled through the slums of Bombay and Madras, I can coexist with people in the worst and filthiest situations making the best of things. I watch them emerge from coal-black, grease-covered, tin sheds wearing starched and ironed white shirts above pressed pants, carrying briefcases, heading out to work. They keep on smiling amidst all the unfairness and abuse. Even beggars who live on the street manage to take long brooms and sweep their patch of sidewalk. And these people with so little keep doing so much. They do what they can.

I love the resilience of us all, the will to live and survive, the grabbing and sucking onto the life force. I love and appreciate my own survival, realizing I was born to fight, but no longer need to. *L'chaim*!

It is only upon leaving India, crossing back over by foot into Nepal, that I finally let myself feel the full pain and joy. As my passport is stamped, I cry for every beggar, cripple, blind man, street urchin, and mother nursing at the side of the road. I cry for their strength and determination. I cry for their resignation, knowing they will never be exposed to the riches and privilege I enjoy. Their entire existence will be spent on these urine-soaked and dung-encrusted streets, rummaging through garbage, begging from tourists, fighting for the chance to earn a living. I cry with such respect and gratitude for the noble souls making it through very difficult times. Mom included.

I can't stop sobbing. Henry is busy at the customs office, and I am waiting with our pedicab driver who has fought off four others to get our luggage into his bicycle cab in order to have our business. He looks quizzically into my eyes. He seems to ask what the matter is, but he can't possibly know. How can a rich American who has it all have any reason to cry? How can anyone cry for someone else's misery? He'd tell me if he could not to worry, as he will work hard and do good in this life so he will come back in even better circumstances. Perhaps as a rich American.

NINE
Seeking "Judi-ism"

The Buddhists say, "No need to take oneself to dusty countries."
What am I doing traveling so far to find my personal "Judi-ism?"
The native American women helped me surrender into listening
to my body, then aging had brought on a deeper surrender to
my body's fallibility. Even though my back pains cleared up after
fully mourning with the Dr. Dash prescriptions, I might still try
"going to the *schwitz*." *Schwitzen* in Yiddish is "to sweat." There
might be a Russian-Jewish way to transcend the body to
find spirit.

Due to dear Grandpa Stockman, who drank himself into a mental
hospital at a time when no Jew acknowledged alcoholism,
having schlepped the steppes of Russia to land at Ellis Island, I
was now privileged to head for the 10th Street Russian baths in
New York City. This historical landmark had, at the turn of the
twentieth century, welcomed the tired bodies of seamstresses,
political pamphleteers, labor organizers, Russian revolutionaries,
and Hassidic housewives seeking relief from cold-water flats,

continuous pregnancies, overwork, and exhaustion. Margaret Sanger, risking death, had provided them with birth control options. Emma Goldman lived around the corner. The Triangle Shirtwaist factory fire happened just a few blocks away. I want to *schwitz* where these women *schwitzed.* I want to mix my juices with theirs.

It's a hike up the white marble steps of this Lower East Side brownstone. It appears at first like you are entering someone's tenement residence. Immediately to the left of the outer entrance is a counter announcing "10TH STREET RUSSIAN BATHS." I'm shocked that a scruffy, bearded, hairy man in tank top with black beret is "manning" the desk on "ladies' day."

The place is jumping with anxious, harried New York women, shrilling out requests for massage appointments. Boris does his best to avoid talking to them while shuffling papers. He doesn't like talking with so many Americans. Native New Yorkers have recently taken over the place. Boris likes taking the D train in from Brighton Beach each day, so he has no need to learn English. All his needs can be met by his neighborhood shopkeepers who also haven't bothered to master the language of their new land. I remember the story of why Grandma Rose had married alcoholic Manual. "He spoke such good English. He was no greenhorn, stumbling to put a sentence together. Spending his days in saloons with those 'Tilaners' gave him an Amurrikun accent." (Every immigrant group had a pejorative term for the other. This was Grandma Rose's reference to Italians who had taught her husband tricks of the street fruit-vendor trade and given him a roadmap to the best watering holes in Philadelphia.)

Broken-English Boris assigns the other ladies their treatments, and I am pushed to the front of the line. First I wonder about the large sign overhead: "Straight Place."

"What does that mean?" I quiz.

"Well, you know." He flaps his right hand back and forth.

"Oh. You mean not gay?"

"Yah, yah. Mit AIDS und alles. Boris the only bath house in New York still open. Vatchoo vant?"

His intense eyes cut like a scalpel straight through me. At the same time, he talks *at* me like I am bothering him and he wants me out of his way as soon as possible. His head jerks back at each utterance, like a drill sergeant ordering troops, "DISS-MISSED."

A slim, talky, petite young thing with a wild hat is joking and gossiping with him while he works. He seems agitated, spouting what I imagine are Russian expletives. Their gossip is about Boris's ex-partner, Ivan, who'd split off on his own and is stealing clients. Wild Hat assures Boris that Ivan's business won't last. "He's only trading off your good reputation." I'm reminded of a childhood watching women cajoling and quieting angry Russian men.

I try to wedge in to gain some information and instruction about their highly recommended *platza* experience.

"What is a *platza*?" I ask meekly.

"Not much time. All gulls busy," Boris barks in a heavy accent. 'You vant massage, *platza,* or just *schvitz*?" He rattles off names of treatments and staff to deliver them, but I am having trouble with his accent, the new names, and the negligible explanations. I know the *platza* involves being beaten with oak branches. Supposed to increase circulation. In some Buddhist sects, head monks beat devotees with a bamboo stick to help them pay closer attention. This is probably the Jewish variation on the bamboo stick–whacking.

Boris is fed up with my hesitation. He points a dismissive finger and barks out *his* decision for me. "You take Black Sea salt massage with Natasha at three and then wait and see if Kira can give you *platza* at four. You just wait. Pay now."

His abruptness stuns me into total silence. His wild-hatted soother friend is full of pep and ready to advise me. "I've been here all day. You must do both treatments."

I place my charge card on the counter and Boris immediately swoops it up while yelling at me when I am confused about the wait for Kira. "Now, will you listen or not? I will only tell if you listen."

I'm slightly embarrassed, but more amused at the Old World style of this little guy. He's abusive, the way my grandfather was with my mother. He makes me into his child, reprimands me for my confusion, and forces me to pay attention. Not the Buddhist gentleness, but my attention is absorbed and riveted.

With piercing eyes, he again points a determined finger and growls out, "Kira best! Can't rush. Overbooked. You have to wait."

No pampering here. My senses awaken to childhood bruisings hearing that guttural Russian accent my grandpa barked at his welfare tenants. As Boris barks more orders, I retire meekly to the ladies' locker room. On the way I pass the "health bar." Instead of spa cuisine canapés or wheat-grass smoothies, the glass refrigerated case doubling as a counter serves up moldy meat, highlighted by large slabs of steaks and corned beef and a grotesque pickled tongue drying on an old leaf of romaine. It's a scene from Conrad's *Heart of Darkness*. "The horror. The horror." Wonder what my Buddhist friends would say about *this*.

Well, enough about flesh. Time for me to join mounds of it in the dressing room. This is no spiffy, clean, chrome-and–glass, modern health spa, with cupboards of fluffy folded towels and pitchers of lemon water stocked by recent immigrants busy wiping countertops. This is instead down and dirty, black Russian. Most prominent in view are successive rows of rusting iron bunk beds, covered with worn flannel sheets atop thin, blue, pinstriped canvas mattresses.

There is a lot of trash on the floor, wrappers off shampoo bottles, hairpins left in sinks, empty toothpaste tubes. Enclosing the beds are brown metal lockers imported from a demolished high school gym somewhere (or perhaps a closed military base). Young Russian "attendants," lounging out on the bunks, are chattering with each other in harsh guttural tones, undoubtedly complaining about working such a hard day. Definitely "old-time religion" here. Amongst these women I'm reminded of my great attraction to the style and dress of the 1940s. It's why I like going to vintage stores to buy old silk slips and tap pants and glass brooches worn by women during the war years. It's my mother's early adult life. It's when Jews were most persecuted. I want to be a part of the trials of these women. I want to be real, under siege.

I undress quickly, putting my things into the wrong locker (I'd later learn). The number on my key does not match the door. No one told me. In fact, no one in authority tells me or anyone else ANYTHING. Where do we find things like towels, robes, where the toilet is? The girls look up from their chatter and point.

Making my way through the locker room, I find a progesterone parade. Women's bodies of all shapes and contours jump into view. No one seems at all concerned about modesty or cover-ups. The heavy velvet curtain that separates us from Boris's front desk keeps flapping in the breeze, mimicking many of the breasts that fall in and out of view. I just want to encircle myself as best I can with the smallish towel provided, and then get downstairs to the *schwitzing* caverns.

Unevenly spaced, steep rock stairs need to be conquered. A short person like myself and the thousands of little old Jewish ladies who've climbed them since 1892 had to be a little unsettled in our rubber flip-flops. I'm sure this precarious descent is getting us ready for surrenders yet to come.

Opening the large, heavy door to "the baths" requires both hands and strong legs and shoulders, and portends further surrender. Nude women sit around the ice-cold pool on benches with their feet up and eyes rolled back. A steam room filled with bodies and an intermittent freezing shower occupy the left. I'm told, "It is a very mild steam room. Nothing like the Russian." A steaming Jacuzzi boils off to the right next to small massage rooms with wet beds. Just past the showers, a sign on a large wooden door announces, "Russian Steam Room."

"Hotter than Hades," according to Boris.

I quickly realize I've brought no toiletries, not even shampoo. Where the hell do I think I am? Spoiled by all the pampering of California "spa" experiences, I'm used to being serviced.

Sorry, baby, no pampering here.

A curly-haired, plump woman who'd stayed there many hours of her life loans me shampoo. She's a regular.

Waiting for showers, I encounter someone who might be sister to the redheaded nose blower who'd aggravated me in the bath cubicle at Shasta Abbey. She's emaciated, appears thirty-five, but starvation and malnutrition certainly could have aged her prematurely. As seven of us line up waiting for the shower, she stands in the stall, curtain flung open, oblivious. She's slowly and meticulously brushing her teeth. No one confronts her. The rawness of the skin on her back attests that she's used to a life of abuse. She's probably much better at enduring pain than we more rounded ladies-in-waiting. We wait some more.

Finally, after showering, I am now cleaned up and ready for Natasha with the Black Sea salt massage.

First, I need further washing. And boy, does she! I am laid out on a foam-covered table and then hosed down with warm, gentle water. Natasha sudses me up and, with deft fingers and loofa brush, massages and scrapes my body. Absolutely heavenly! No way can you escape feeling body beautiful. She gives artful attention everywhere she touches. Without a doubt I've found my true calling. Definitely "to the manner born."

Nina, short for Ninotchka, joins Natasha and they lift me up and gently guide me toward the large Russian steam room. In broken English, Natasha explains, "Russian bath better than Turkish bath. Larger and, oh my got, hotter."

I wonder if it reaches sweat lodge numbers?

It takes a half second in the steam room to find out. Definitely "Oh my got! Hottttterrrrr."

My eyes squint into the heat. There are three tiers of wide stairs covered with wooden planks ascending to the concrete ceiling. Down from this ceiling, massive furnaces pipe out heat, heat, and more heat. At each level of stairs five faucets run continuously, emptying into beige plastic buckets overflowing with icy-cold water. These plastic pails empty incessantly, cascading down to each lower tier with a constant meditative drip. Acclimatizing and working to keep my breathing shallow, I watch others to see what to do. Various nude or scantily clad bodies saunter over to pick up these pails and empty the full contents over their heads. The pails quickly refill for more dousing. Did I mention yet it's really, really hot?

The room is truly magnificent. The large, cut rocks were assembled by hand, like the Inca ruins in Peru. From the three tiers of landings, nude women *schwitz,* gazing down to the center ring where a large wooden table sits, covered with a mat and wet towels for Kira's *platza* treatments. At this Roman forum, all senators peer down while continuing their own personal dousings, wrappings of heads in washcloths, or laying out of limbs.

I sit down slowly onto the bottom tier of boards, realizing that the higher you go, the hotter it gets. I take in my first glimpse of Kira. Early twenties, wears cotton panties rolled down and up, making them into a bikini with a thong ass. Nothing on top, great figure, wears a ring in her nose. I can only think how hot that ring must get after so many hours in that steam room. Her hair is tousled, dirty blonde, and she tries to keep it tied up.

It's grueling to watch her work on a fragile-looking blonde woman on the table. And work she does, really getting into the sensuality and the rhythm of things. She closes her eyes and seems to pick up her subject's aura. She massages the body while rhythmically breathing and pushing with her whole being. Beside the table sit two gigantic, soapy buckets filled with bound clusters of oak leaves. At timed intervals during the massage, Kira stops, picks up these bunches, and beats the fragile blonde about the shoulders, buttocks, and back. She stops to take a break, to get a cooling shower for herself. Before exiting, she turns the lady over, placing one *platza* on her breasts and another on her pubic bone, and quickly leaves the room.

I'm petrified as well as excited about my upcoming debut. I know I have to experience this thing, but there is a wait. It's clear that appointment times mean nothing, and Boris neglects to tell anyone that they might end up waiting until late into the evening.

Does he care that I have a later appointment? He has the credit card imprint. The curly-haired shampoo lady assures me it's worth waiting for. Yeah, but she stays in the *schwitz* for hours, never taking a break. She can handle this. I might die.

I decide to occupy myself by further evaluating bodies. There are two black women with stylish, Native-style beads around their waists, just a few bulbous-stomached old Black Sea women, and countless young women with very hairy pubes.

Each time Kira takes a break, I let her know I'm waiting, that I've importantly "just flown in from the coast," that I am scared and anxious and have an early dinner date.

Eventually Kira is ready for me. She gives me the high sign and points to the table. The Greek chorus is assembled, and I lie down on my stomach as instructed. The stifling air makes breathing difficult, and I know now I'm petrified with good cause. Kira begins a slow massage, but quickly moves to the beating. The pounding heaviness of those clumps of leaves is much more than I'd bargained for.

Better than a bamboo rod from a Buddhist monk? Less painful than a hot poker in the eye? Well, yes, but . . .

I know I'm probably going to die. Instead I breathe into it, heaving a sigh with each blow while my body oozes into limpness. Kira plops me over on my back, slams the branches onto my chest and pubes, and leaves for her break. My breathing is slowing down when she returns. As she resumes the massage, my shoulders heave and flow into her hands. She pulls on my arms and my whole body follows. She owns me. I'm a limp dishrag. I have no sense of time or place. *What dinner date?* It's just me and her and the heat. It's just heat, trying to breathe, praying to survive, and the heat. Instead of reaching for a feared ice-cold bucket, I ask Kira to splash me. Otherwise, I'm sure I'll pass out. She picks up the pail and *whoosh,* its contents cover us both. We smile.

I surrender. Strangely, the cold blast is not a shock. My pulsating, overdone body stops baking and begins cooling, and I breathe without panic. I'm emptied of all my brilliant ideas and open to receiving whatever she has to offer.

When Kira resumes the beating/massage, she stands above my protruding tush and begins a long, smooth swoosh from my buttocks to my shoulders. When she gets near my head, she stops, her body leaning over mine, her voice low at my ear.

"Body responsive," she coos in an almost unintelligible Russian accent.

"No need think. Body good worker. Strong body. Heavy legs."

She then moves lower, wraps herself around my gargantuan, solid-rock thighs, holding one hand over the top, the other on the bottom, and coos, "Good *pulkas*. Good worker. Let body let goooooo." She quickly pulls back to full standing, digging the base of her palms down my back. Once again she swooshes up to my ear and continues.

This time she turns my face toward hers and I focus on the glint from that golden nose ring, feeling her breath coming out of each nostril.

"Must be strong, like body. Do what life instruct. Follow *pulkas*. Get all out of here."

She then stands up, grabs the *platza,* and heavily pounds my full torso and legs.

I'm lost in contemplating my *pulkas*. *Don't our thighs house the strongest muscles of the body? Am I not fit as a fiddle but still carry gigunda pulkas? If that's where I hold the excess weight, might that be where I hold my strength to escape the loony bin? So I'm slightly overweight. It's a lot of muscle.*

I suffer from what Naomi Wolf calls the "One Stone Solution." A stone in British measurement equals fourteen US pounds. She says that's what all American women want to lose. *Are my* pulkas *my extra fourteen pounds?*

The next thing I hear is "FINISH! NEXT!" as Kira ignores me, looking around for her next customer.

It's over much too quickly. I smile weakly and hobble out to the cooler shower room. Kira yells to my retreating back, "You must jump into pool. Right away or you pass out." I settle my lobster-red skin right down into the icy pool. It doesn't hurt. Actually, I feel nothing at all.

I then plop onto a bench and stare blankly at all the other nudies lined up for showers, tying hair up in towels, or smearing themselves with body scrubs.

Dazed and limp, I'm back to body watching. With clay packs on their faces, they all look like scruffy Daryl Hannah in that movie *The Clan of the Cave Bear. I wonder if those primitives weren't really doing facials*. They're all like the ladies in Burma smeared with *Tanaka* clay. Universal oneness?

As I rest, four different women approach to comment on my *platza* massage. In a nutshell: "Watching the two of you was an unbelievable experience. There was something highly spiritual going on. Your ordeal was so different from the others. You seemed to surrender to her, to give it all up. She seemed to sense that and really gave to you. You were both more into the joint experience than into yourselves or each other."

Just like in tango.

None of these observers noticed that Kira spoke to me. I wonder if she really did. *What did she mean by "get all out of here?" Did she mean for me to get her out? Was she sold into slavery? Did she mean for me to get myself out, get the Russian out of my system? Did she mean all women need to stop primping for men, stop worrying about their bodies? Did she mean we were all being stifled? What did she mean about trusting the strong body and the good-worker* pulka *legs?*

As I look around at other short, big-legged Russian women, I see clearly what a hardship I must have been to my mother. The things that brought many mothers pride about their daughters were things that further alienated us. I had chosen a different life. Like Kira advised, I'd spent my life *getting out.* I lived with the normies, "passed" in good company.

Somehow, I don't feel guilty anymore. I'd followed my *pulkas* and it was okay to be out of the muck and mire.

Dressing without thinking, I know I don't want to leave the place. I want my nap on the rusting iron bunks. I want to keep watching women come and go.

Combing my hair over the cracked sink, I see a shadowy reflection: my mom's face in the mirror.

Why is she here?

Is she telling me it's okay for me to leave?

She's handing me a ticket out. It's okay.

Checking out with Boris is just as disorganized as the check-in, but he's much less insulting. I guess I've had my trial by fire and he respects me for it. He's busy issuing membership cards at the counter. He makes these himself, first snapping Polaroid pictures of new members and then pasting a square of yellow legal paper to the back where he'll record each of their visits. Nothing very high-tech and modern. He notices me watching, smiles, and says with a twinkle, "Nothing fencey."

His comment says it all about the place and the experience, but also says a lot about my journey. These are my roots. Nothing fancy. I come from horror, filth, abuse, and ultimate survival. Forged by fire, my strong, grounded thighs will lead me out. I can't leave the fat self behind. I can't deny my own dark side. I can accept everyone else as well. Even Mom. And I can have compassion for all those bulimics, appearing so perfect on the outside, who hide black garbage bags filled with puke in large mounds in the backs of bedroom closets. I walk back out into the cold New York winter, passing dope dealers huddled on stoops at St. Mark's Place. I am filled with gratitude. I love my mother and her conflicts. Instead of the previous revulsion, I understand the struggle, the survival, the grappling with life. I even appreciate the filth. I have all choices available. I feel like the great therapist Harry Stack Sullivan, who said, "Nothing human is foreign to me." I can channel high class or low down and love it all freely and gratefully.

TEN
You're Here Now

I wouldn't return to the abbey for several years. I really didn't even want to. Becoming more secure in my personal life, accepting the waning of my media work, feeling like I have less and less to teach others, I settle in. Henry retires and we set up permanent residence in Palm Springs. With a few exceptions, public speaking and audiences are totally off my radar screen. I lecture regularly at the Betty Ford Center, a twenty-minute drive from my desert retreat, consult for a new spa resort a five-minute bike ride away, and accept whatever traveling lecture gigs sound fun and beneficial. I also love the phone coaching. Without the visuals, I rely on other senses and find connections with people thousands of miles away who are willing to be more intimate on the phone than face-to-face. Happy my back pain has subsided, and appreciating the lives my phone clients share with me, I am content. With tango, I balance on gigantic, rock-solid, oh-so-functional thighs! I love them.

The abbey seems so very far away. But I know I have to go back. I know it will help to have a few minutes in that environment of honesty and authenticity. I long to just sit there and meditate.

Reverend Kincaid finally answers the phone. His accent doesn't seem quite as New York. The lilting giggle is still there. "Judi, I'm so sorry, but we are closed for the winter, accepting no visitors."

I beg, "Please, I just want to spend a little time there. I really need it. I can just walk around and won't bother anyone, maybe meditate a little?"

Still the special-case scenario.

"Well, okay, but there will be no program for you."

I don't care.

Snowstorms are quickly descending on Grants Pass, so I can only visit the abbey, at the most, for two hours, and then have to get on my way.

"You won't be able to take meals or pray with the monks. All are on special retreat. Maybe you can just sit and listen to a tape in the guest house."

"Whatever. I just want to be on the grounds. It's such a safe house for me."

"Okay," he counters and then hangs up.

Reverend Hoko, whom I've never met, greets me at the still-wobbly metal gate, accepting my proffered poinsettia plant.

She greets me solemnly, with no smile. "Since there is no one currently available to show you around the grounds, you are welcome to sit in the guest house meditation hall. The main *zendo* and other buildings are locked."

"I'm fine. I really have no preferences."

Well, to be truthful, I'd love to see Reverend Kincaid. Well, to be really truthful, I want to be in the zendo, *want to sit in the cemetery, want, want, want.*

I'm led to the meditation room beside the entrance to the new guest house. Before facing my chair toward the wall, I notice a blustering light snowfall amongst the pines.

I'm home.

I sit for an hour, then take a ten-minute walking meditation break. As I settle in to resume, Reverend Hoko whispers by my ear, "Judi, may I please talk with you outside?" Oddly enough, though I'd faintly heard the door open, I'm startled by her soft, soothing voice. She smiles and leaves to wait for me out in the anteroom.

She must have talked with someone, as her manner is quite different. "You've been with us before?"

I explain my other visits.

Careful, Jude, you're starting into a qualifying-exam mode.

"I suppose it will be okay for you to wander the grounds by yourself, then."

I nod and bow appreciatively.

She outlines which areas will be off-limits to my wanderings. "The monks are assured privacy in some parts of the cloisters. When you are ready to leave, we will get someone to unlock the gate."

We both bow.

My old cemetery spot is off-limits this trip. She recommends the "pet cemetery," her personal favorite. I head there first, but as the wind and snow flurries are kicking up, I quickly move under cover to wander the cloisters. The roofs are protecting rows and rows of stacked firewood.

Like Boy Scouts, these monks; ever ready and prepared.

As I round the corner by the back dining hall steps, I recall the orange peel incident. There stands Reverend Kincaid, chatting with another monk!

He quickly approaches, pointing at his chest. "Hi, Judi. Reverend Kincaid, in case you don't recognize me."

I bow *gassho*.

How could I forget that smile?

"I'll walk with you for a bit if you like."

Would I like?

"I guess I can even take you into the *zendo* as I have a key."

All my wants delivered, and I don't even pray to get them.

As we walk, it's obvious I've forgotten all the important bowing points on the path. I follow his lead.

Neither of us misses a beat as he leads, bows, and keeps up a steady stream of conversation. I guess when it's not retreat time, they talk more. He's catching me up on all the news.

"We've had vandalism. Reverend Kinnett has just died. I've been back to New York a few times to visit my parents."

I feel much more equal and whole with him. I don't need to audition. I'm happy I don't try to explain how much I live by Buddhist precepts today without even trying.

The initial deprivations learned at Shasta Abbey developed for me later defenses against compulsive eating. I now often easily leave a last string bean on my plate, and say no to yet another pistachio nut. Sometimes I even have perspective around a slice of dark chocolate cake. I give it one LUST look. Not one "last" look, but one "lust" look. I've learned about *preference* versus *insistence.* When I can take it or leave it, then I can have it. However, when in lust mode, one bite is too many and a thousand isn't enough. I decide to postpone it for later when my pulse isn't racing, when my mouth isn't salivating, when I can be in a state of calm and equanimity. I learned about that calm, "equanimous" state at the abbey.

I trust my body to let me know. The body doesn't lie. My head can talk me into anything, but my body will signal what's out of sync. Lately my body shuns beef. I've become a vegephile, craving veggies!

I'd love to tell him how his loving kindness and encouragement comforted my fear and allowed me to stay. Clearly, only warmth and caring can motivate surrender. If your kid's oatmeal dries on the table, it is like concrete to remove. If you try to chip away at it, you will take the finish off your furniture. If you take a warm, moist facecloth and just lay it on top, the oatmeal will slowly melt and dissolve, becoming easy to wipe away.

I'd love to tell him how gentle awareness and trust developed slowly over time. But he knows all about it. Buddhists describe this gentle transformation by comparing it to walking through a foggy, misty day. Without even realizing it, you come out the other side of the fog fully drenched.

It is the same type of gradual, progressive change that happens while growing into a full-blown eating disorder. No one notices when crossing lines from moderation to excessive use to addictive obsession. A deli grocer might ask, "When does a cucumber soaked in brine become a pickle?" In spiritual surrender, I've gradually shed obsessive behavior and moved toward the spiritual, moderate, middle path.

I guess you get pickled into the spiritual dimension whether you ask for it or not.

I'd found that personal middle path by first careening through center like a trapeze flyer swinging from bar to bar. Each time I'd glimpse center in an over-the-shoulder glance to see what a moderate, centered place looked like. Becoming more familiar with center, as the pendulum stopped swinging so violently, slowly plopping to midpoint, I could settle into a familiar place I'd sailed through a few thousand times before.

I'd love to show him even more how the concepts I learned here have carried back into my real world. Instead, now I am the one practicing that verbal economy, and I just listen.

Before leaving, though, I tell him about my travels in India and that I've been to Malaysia, to the temple where Reverend Kinnett received her ordination. I explain excitedly how the monk there even gave me an acupuncture treatment for my back pain. I feel safe enough to ask him, "Why do they practice Buddhism so differently than what I see at the abbey? In Asia, they go into these temples with incense they call joss sticks and throw them down, like with the *I Ching,* to divine their fortunes. It feels like a gaming hall with very little attention to spirit or reverence. Temples seem like casinos. Even though they bow reverently, everyone seems there just to place their bets."

"You experienced the difference between at-home practice and religion for export," he answers. "Most dogmas are not as reverently held at home. When Westerners experienced the essence of Buddhism, that is what they extracted to take home. A lot of the holiness of the practice is taken for granted in Asia."

And all my accomplishments were not revered at home, either by me or my mother. Maybe it was all just taken for granted. And that might be why I could accept the spiritual path more easily in Asia, as it was something each lives without comment. No one philosophized, or at least that is what I understood. It was more funky, smelly, down-to-earth . . . just like home.

At that great, heavy temple door, Reverend Kincaid unlocks a large metal padlock and we're in the *zendo,* dark as usual.

"It seems so much smaller than I remember it."

"Perhaps you have become bigger, more fully present in yourself."

He shows me the current monks' quarters, which will soon accommodate future lay trainees. I'm seeing into the inner workings, viewing things that had previously been forbidden. I see how the monks manage to squeeze bed linens, and all their earthly belongings, into a very small cubicle.

We saunter over to an altar. It houses a dead cat, waiting for later burial. Reverend Kincaid shares with me, "His brother is going to be so lonely. They've been inseparable, constant companions."

Soon, it's time for me to go. Again at the chicken-wire gate, I stammer and cry.

"It's . . . been so important for me. . . . to have this visit. It is so important for me that you are here." I'm remembering that monks in Tibet take shifts continuously meditating, believing their effort is saving the planet.

"As long as you are here, it enables me to continue out there."

He smiles with eyes shining, that widened, childlike, Zen thing.

I bow to him and to the rickety gate as I leave. My eyes are now wide too.

Driving away, I hear echoes of Reverend Muldoon.

"When the bowing dies, Buddhism dies . . . ."

EPILOGUE

Bloom Where You're Planted

More than a decade after Mom's death, we are escaping the desert heat with a summer stay in New York City. I am able to drive into Brooklyn without shaking or feeling sick. My mind has made friends with my body and I am content to be a comfortable, sensuous woman. I usually eat moderately, often using Divine Dine techniques I learned at the abbey. Food is rarely an issue. It has assumed a proper place in my life, used for nurturance, not punishment. Are these results permanent? Is anything?

I regularly bike, swim, and dance. With yoga thrown in, my back doesn't hurt. Now, the knee, that's another story. At a recent visit to my orthopedist to examine MRI results, he looked up from the pictures in astonishment and said, "I don't see how you are walking. With your left knee and right ankle, you really don't have a leg to stand on. According to these tests, you should be crawling in here wailing with pain. Whatever you're doing, I recommend you keep it up." He should only know what a spiritual inside job it is to keep the structural integrity. And what is holding me up? In addition to daily soulful surrender . . . those giant, heavy-duty, doing-double-duty *thighs*!

It's the Fourth of July, the streets are teeming, and parking doesn't exist. A barricade is set up across Brighton's 15th Street, but a family is loading beach chairs into a large SUV parked right in front of Mom's building.

They are, in fact, leaving, as the driver jokes, "How much you willing to pay for the space?"

It's right in front of her building!

I have no palpitations. I am no longer a bad seed, nor have I sprouted from a rotten plant. We've been weeded.

It turns out to be a perfect New York City day, looking at junk, watching the haggling with street vendors. I encounter a statuesque, quintessential New York woman with white T-shirt and a pretty beige linen rendition of slacks I have been seeking all over the city: wide-legged, high-waisted, newly recycled fashion from the seventies. I follow her halfway across the street and interrupt her stride with "Please excuse me, but I've been looking everywhere for slacks like those. Could you tell me where you found them?"

She smiles a wry grin and answers, "I got these in California."

"Where?"

"In Palm Springs, on sale."

"You're kidding! I live in Palm Springs."

"They're at the Armani store at the Cabazon outlet mall."

Mmmmmm? You mean it's all in my own backyard? I feel like Dorothy at the end of *The Wizard of Oz*.

Farther down the boardwalk, I stop at a bench overlooking the ocean. As all those Russian voices loom up in that staccato, guttural chatter, nothing wrenches inside me. Even the English speakers, complaining or bragging about daughters, sons, or grandchildren, no longer ignite a fever. The spell has lifted; just calm air around my body. Watching people in beach attire lugging paraphernalia, crossing at the light . . . above and around it all, from radio speakers, a familiar, husky-voiced Louis Armstrong croons about it being a wonderful world.

Viewing the passing crowd, I realize they'll all die someday, and a new crop will move in to line up at the beach. And I'll be gone too. Mom and I and all those beachgoers crossing at the light have just a few years here. We pay attention to traffic laws and then each find our own way across. If only we can keep our eyes open and enjoy.

I reach the famous Nathan's hot dog stand at Coney Island to hear a blaring announcement: "The United States must win back its famous Independence Day title!" The Japanese Takeru Kobayashi has held the world championship of Nathan's hot dog-eating contest for six full years.

Kobayashi, at 165 pounds, has been announcing all week to the International Federation of Competitive Eating that he has a "sports injury," arthritis of the jaw, but will compete anyway.

At six-foot-six and 230 pounds, Joey Chestnut, our great red, white, and blue hope, is, at twenty-three years old, returning from California to take back our honor.

"We're 50,000 strong here today," bellows the announcer sporting straw hat and bowtie, revving up the balloon–and–banner-waving crowd. It's a gray, foggy day at the beach, but the crowd's enthusiasm is not at all dampened. They're playing for the international TV cameras, yelling enthusiastically for our hope, our champ . . . "Joe-eee, Joe-eee, Joe-eee."

It's a gut-busting showdown, combining drama, daring, and indigestion. With veins extended on his forehead, downing sixty-six hot dogs, including buns, in twelve minutes, Joey takes back our eating supremacy! As he accepts the mustard-yellow belt, he manages to utter a full-throated "It's about time the championship came home. If I needed to eat another one right now, I could."

Love Dogs

by Rumi

One night a man was crying,
Allah! Allah!
His lips grew sweet with the praising,
until a cynic said,
"So! I have heard you
calling out, but have you ever
gotten any response?"

The man had no answer to that.
He quit praying and fell into a confused sleep.
He dreamed he saw Khidr, the guide of souls,
in a thick, green foliage.

"Why did you stop praising?"
"Because I've never heard anything back."

"This longing you express
is the return message."

The grief you cry out from
draws you toward union.

Your pure sadness
that wants help
is the secret cup.

Listen to the moan of a dog for its master.
That whining is the connection.

There are love dogs
no one knows the names of.

Give your life to be one of them.

Other Materials by Dr. Judi Hollis

BOOKS
- *Fat Is a Family Affair* (Harper/Hazelden)
- *Fat & Furious* (Ballantine)
- *Hot & Heavy* (Health Communications, Inc.)
- *It's Not a Dress Rehearsal* (HOLSEM Productions)
- *Let Them Eat Cake* (HOLSEM Productions)

PAMPHLETS
- "Accepting Powerlessness" (Hazelden)
- "Relapse for Easting Disorder Sufferers" (Hazelden)
- "Resisting Recovery" (Hazelden)
- "When AA's Go to OA" (Hazelden)
- "Humility vs. Humiliation" (Hazelden)
- "Transferring Obsessions" (Hazelden)
- "I'm Not Ready Yet" (Hazelden)

VIDEOS
- "Family Matters" (Hazelden Foundation)
  Dick Young Productions, New York City
- "Dark Secrets, Bright Victory" (Hazelden Foundation)
  Dick Young Productions, New York City
- "Dignity Dine" (HOLSEM Productions)
- "Live to Eat-Eat to Live" (HOLSEM Productions)
- "Starving for Perfection" (HOLSEM Productions)

CDS
- "Hope for Compulsive Overeaters," Vols. 1 & 2 (Hazelden)
- "Fat Is a Family Affair" (Hazelden)
- "Codependent Compulsions" (HOLSEM Productions)
- "Y2 OA?" (HOLSEM Productions)
- "Let's Talk Radio" (HOLSEM Productions)
- "Going Deep" (HOLSEM Productions)
- "Fat & Furious" (HOLSEM Productions)

For ordering or more information about videos, audios, CDs, DVDs, books, and seminars, please call 800-8-ENOUGH or go to www.JUDIHOLLIS.com.